Praise from Health Professionals

"I highly recommend the Metabolic Nutrition program to every
healthcare professional looking for a way to offer a unique, easy,
and affordable tool for greater health and well-being for their practice.
I had read about and purchased other metabolic profiling systems
previously, but, they were too difficult, confusing, and expensive to be
practical. This one just makes sense, is based on sound science, and
is very user-friendly for both practitioner and client."
　　　—Sue Ryno, R.N., N.P., Ph.D.

"Metabolic Typing is the answer to, and the missing link for, my
nutritional practice. I would encourage anyone in the medical field to
seriously consider incorporating Metabolic Typing into their practice."
　　　—Bryan W. Barry, D.C.

"I had an interest in Metabolic Typing before, but now have a passion for
it! I think that every health practitioner needs this information."
　　　—Tara Jeffery, R.N.

"I have been using Dr. Kristal's Metabolic Typing program for
approximately five years with fantastic results. Almost all my patients
report increased energy and a reduction in many symptoms when
they stick to their individualized diet. It is especially effective for chronic
fatigue, fibromyalgia, and autoimmune disorders. I am very impressed
with the results. Many of my patients have been able to reduce or
eliminate their prescription meds while on the program. I would highly
recommend Dr. Kristal's Metabolic Typing program. You will be amazed
by the results."
　　　—John Sherman, N.D.

"I have a Masters Degree and I'm a Doctor of Chiropractic, but, despite
my education, I couldn't control my blood sugar problems very well.
Once I learned my Metabolic Type and began to eat accordingly,
my previous low blood sugar problems vanished."
　　　—John Harrington, D.C.

"All those who wish to be as healthy as they can be, and especially those with health problems that defy conventional treatments, should read this book."
—John R. Lee, M.D.

Individual Testimonials

"I have not had an illness since I began the regimen, not even a cold, while at the same time, people around me seem to be catching viruses all the time."
—GB

"A tremendous *quality of life* change has occurred since I discovered Metabolic Typing. I am sixty-one years old, but two years ago I thought I was dying. I was very sick then, but I'm not sick now!"
—DB

"In eight weeks I have lost twenty-two pounds; but it is not the weight that I have lost that makes me feel so good; it's the food that I now eat that gives me so much energy. I feel fabulous."
—LM

"My family and I are so grateful for your help. Many thanks for the good health. What a gift you are giving!"
—AR

"Following the Metabolic Typing program has literally changed my life! My presenting problem was stomach difficulties, which my HMO doctor was unable to diagnose or relieve. But now, with my special diet and supplements, I am symptom free, have lost twenty pounds, and feel great."
—KC

"One doesn't often meet someone who is so genuinely passionate about their work, and is so willing to reach out and help others. Thank you Dr. Kristal."
—LQ

THE NUTRITION SOLUTION

A Guide to
Your Metabolic Type

Harold J. Kristal, D.D.S.
&
James M. Haig, N.C.

North Atlantic Books
Berkeley, California

Published by   Book design by Jennifer Dunn
North Atlantic Books   Cover design by Paula Morrison
P.O. Box 12327
Berkeley, California 94712   Printed in the United States of America

The Nutrition Solution: A Guide to Your Metabolic Type is sponsored by the Society for the Study of Native Arts and Sciences, a nonprofit educational corporation whose goals are to develop an educational and crosscultural perspective linking various scientific, social, and artistic fields; to nurture a holistic view of arts, sciences, humanities, and healing; and to publish and distribute literature on the relationship of mind, body, and nature.

North Atlantic Books are available through most bookstores. To contact North Atlantic directly, call (800) 337-2665 or visit our website at www.northatlanticbooks.com.

Substantial discounts on bulk quantities of North Atlantic books are available to corporations, professional associations, and other organizations. For details and discount information, contact the special sales department at North Atlantic Books.

LIBRARY OF CONGRESS CATALOGING-IN-PUBLICATION DATA

Kristal, Harold J., 1925–
    The nutrition solution : a guide to your metabolic type / by Harold Kristal with James Haig.
        p. cm.
    Includes bibliographical references and index.
        ISBN 1-55643-437-5 (pbk.)
    1. Nutrition. 2. Metabolism. 3. Phenotype. 4. Diet in disease. 5. Diet therapy.
I. Haig, James M., 1951– II. Title.
    RA784 .K75 2002
    613'.2—dc21

                                                                      2002015093

            1   2   3   4   5   6   7   /   06   05   04   03   02

This book is dedicated to my clients,
to all practitioners of Metabolic Typing,
and to everyone
who seeks better health through nutrition.

A Note on the Use of the Personal Pronoun and Proper Names

Please note that whenever the personal pronoun "I" is used in this book, it refers to the principal author, Harold J. Kristal. Also, the names used in the case histories have been changed to preserve the privacy of the individuals involved.

Disclaimer

The information contained in this book is for educational purposes only. It is not intended to be used to diagnose or treat any disease, and is not a substitute or a prescription for proper medical advice, intervention, or treatment. Any consequences resulting from the application of this information will be the sole responsibility of the reader. Neither the authors nor the publisher will be liable for any damage caused, or alleged to be caused, by the application of the information in this book. Individuals with a known or suspected health condition are strongly encouraged to seek the advice of a licensed healthcare professional before implementing any of the protocols in this book.

Acknowledgments

This book would not have been possible without the encouragement and support of many people. I would especially like to thank my co-author and editor James Haig, a fine nutritionist, writer, and Metabolic Typing practitioner in his own right; Liz Paniagua, Marina James, and Vernon Philpott for holding down the fort; Ken Malik for keeping his hand on the tiller, and for his many helpful suggestions for the book; Gael Philpott for her sharp proofreading eyes; my clients for keeping up the pressure to get the book written; and my family for their love and support. I would also like to thank the staff at North Atlantic Books—especially Brooke Warner, Paula Morrison, and Richard Grossinger—for skillfully guiding us through the publishing process. Thanks also to Robert Jay Rowen, M.D., Richard Kunin, M.D., Gabriel Cousens, M.D., Parris Kidd, Ph.D., Edward Winger, M.D., Stephen Levine, Ph.D., and Jeffrey Lioon for their help and input in various ways over the years; to Richard Cristdahl, O.M.D., L.Ac. for contributing to the menu suggestions; and Leni Felton, Louise Dunlap, and Jessica Lewis for their assistance in earlier writing projects. A special thanks to Steven William Fowkes, biochemist, author, and graphic artist, for his wonderful Steroid Tree and all the other illustrations in the book, and for his peerless technical assistance and advice. Thanks also to Joan Lindley for her dedication and perseverance in introducing Metabolic Typing to the UK, and to Alison Loftus and her group of English MT practitioners for carrying the torch. I would also like to thank the many dedicated scientists and clinicians whose own work inspired me, and contributed—directly or indirectly—to my own. Finally, special thanks to John R. Lee, M.D. for his generous Foreword; to Dr. Etienne Callebout for contributing the article on cancer and Metabolic Typing that appears in the Appendix; to the late Adelle Davis for getting me started on the road of nutrition; and to William L. Wolcott, whose genius and inspiration helped all the pieces fall into place.

Table of Contents

List of Illustrations

Chapter 5

Appendix

Foreword

It is well known that conventional medicine is not at its best when counseling patients about nutrition and diet. Standard diets are often handed out, and if they do not seem to suffice, the patients may be referred to a dietitian. Though common sense dictates that nutrition plays a big role in health matters, the underlying metabolic complexity of nutrition is a bit beyond what is offered in most medical schools. Not too long ago, my alma mater, the University of Minnesota Medical School, announced the hiring of two research-oriented nutritional scientists who would be obligated to provide three hours of nutritional education yearly to the medical students. This is just not good enough.

Throughout my medical career, since 1955, I have invested much time and energy in attempting to learn more about nutrition, not only for the sake of my patients' health but also because I recognized my own lack of knowledge of this important subject. I am attracted to puzzle-solving. Looking back over the years, I see that most of the insightful and valuable nutrition books were written not by medical doctors, but by biochemists and, of all people, dentists. I recall, for instance, such wonderful books as *Nutrition Against Disease* and *The Wonderful World Within You* by Roger J. Williams, Ph.D., professor of chemistry at the University of Texas, and director of the Clayton Foundation Biochemical Institute. It was he who first emphasized biological individuality and the need to consider individual metabolic profiles, rather than to speak in terms of a conjectured normal or average person.

Even prior to Professor Williams, there was Adelle Davis, with biochemistry degrees from Purdue, Columbia, and the University of Southern California. Despite these solid credentials, her message of healthful nutritional modification was ignored by conventional medicine or, worse, scorned. In the three-plus decades since she wrote *Let's Eat Right to Keep Fit* and her other popular books, wise clinicians now recognize her message as prescient, authoritative, and important.

The book that stands out for me was *Predictive Medicine: A Study in Strategy,* by Emmanuel Cheraskin and W. M. Ringsdorf, both dentists and professors of Oral Medicine at the Medical Center, University of Alabama. That book was the first to posit that signs and symptoms of disease are merely the outer manifestations of an underlying metabolic, chemical, hormonal, and enzyme imbalance, the key for which is diet. It is clear, I think, that the oral cavity is a mirror of the state of health of the rest of the body. The more progressive dentists understand this.

Other great teachers with whom I have had some personal experience include: Professor Linus Pauling, through his leadership role in the Ortho-molecular Health-Medicine Society in San Francisco; leading alternative medicine pioneers Drs. Jonathan Wright and Alan Gaby; and biochemist Jeffrey Bland, Ph.D., through his wonderful seminars. The talent of these people to draw us into the molecular world of metabolic processes is simply awesome.

In my own years of family practice it did not take long for me to recognize that an ounce of prevention is indeed far better than a pound of treatment; but, furthermore, that finding and treating the underlying cause of an illness is far superior to merely treating its symptoms. There are golden moments in my practice that stand out forever in my memory: when, for example, I suddenly realized that a man with incoordination and odd tingling in his extremities had pernicious anemia (despite having normal red blood cells), and could be cured by monthly injections of vitamin B-12.

In another golden moment, I remember an overweight sixty-five-year-old woman (who could never lose weight by dieting) rather suddenly developing congestive heart failure that was unresponsive to diuretics and other drugs prescribed by her cardiologist. Her husband hinted to me that she was a closet alcoholic. In a split second, I realized that her weight problem was caused by the calories from the vodka she consumed, and that the strict diet she was on created the likelihood of "wet" beri-beri (vitamin B-1 deficiency). I instructed the hospital nurse to add a hefty dose of B-1 to the patient's IV, and the heart failure disappeared within twenty-four hours.

When we moved to Sebastopol twenty-six years ago, our neighbor was a forty-year-old man in good health, except for a painful hip caused by a work accident several years before that forced him to walk with a pronounced limp and left him unable to work. His X-rays showed severe degenerative changes in the cartilage of the hip joint, and numerous orthopedists told him there was no treatment except for hip replacement. However, he was reluctant to accept that judgment. I showed him an article in the *JAMA* illustrating the potential benefit of vitamin C to damaged cartilage. He added four grams of vitamin C daily, and in about three months his hip pain disappeared, and he was able to return to work. Nutrients are powerful things.

In the past two decades, our knowledge of intracellular metabolism has progressed enormously. Medical research, once confined to superficial signs and symptoms, has penetrated, first, the organs and major systems, then cellular activities, and is now deep into intracellular functions such as the mitochondria, cytokines, hormones, and electron transfer. Understanding the mechanisms by which vital nutrients, as well as toxins, do their work is within our reach. But the logarithmic expansion of scientific knowledge has outrun the ability of conventional clinicians to absorb it all. Our peculiar and antiquated practice of specialization by body organs, rather than basing our practice on underlying metabolic concepts, is now recognized as a handicap to true understanding. The newer research now spans the previous gaps between organs and organ systems. A cardiologist may study the effect of magnesium on the heart muscle, but misses its effects elsewhere in the body. Research based on single factors falls by the wayside in the wake of multifactorial realities. The world of medical knowledge has entered a new stage, highly technical and full of complexity. There are leaders among us who grasp these new realities—and we should be paying attention to them. One such leader is Harold J. Kristal.

Harold Kristal practiced dentistry in the San Francisco Bay Area for many years, and I first met him in the early 1970s. His intelligence and enthusiastic grasp of the underlying factors in metabolic matters of health and disease were apparent to all who knew him. Over the years, I referred patients to Dr. Kristal to take advantage of his intellect and his extensive knowledge of metabolic balance. I recall a man in his forties who had severe osteoporosis that had mystified the various top orthopedists he had consulted. I referred him to Dr. Kristal, who, by examining his saliva pH, soon diagnosed the problem as metabolic acidosis and determined that the problem was related to nutrition. However, the usual diet of alkaline vegetables, which customarily buffers acidosis, somehow, if paradoxically, increased the acidosis in this patient. Through trial and error, or perhaps by intuition aided by previous experience, Dr. Kristal found the diet that brought the man's pH back to normal. By following the suggested diet, his osteoporosis reversed and he regained his strong bones. I like to think that incidents such as these were the stimuli that directed Dr. Kristal to his present work, which has culminated in the writing of his remarkable new book, *The Nutrition Solution: A Guide to Your Metabolic Type.*

The premise of the book is simple: Dr. Kristal uses the testing procedures he has developed to find the individual's Metabolic Type; to identify the underlying metabolic problem; and to correct it with nutrition. Balance is the key, and the serum pH is the guide. Optimal total health is the result of optimal cellular health, and in this Dr. Kristal has shown that nutrition is paramount. All people are biologically different, and any given nutrient may have opposite effects in different individuals. The trick is to find the right nutritional solution for each person. Dr. Kristal found a way to make this strategy both possible and effective. He has spent years studying the two great engines of energy—the Oxidative and the Autonomic systems—and their correlation with serum pH and nutritional balance. He has learned the importance of identifying four Metabolic Types—Fast and Slow Oxidizers, and Sympathetics and Parasympathetics—and his work has culminated in a sophisticated but practical program for restoring optimal health.

Now Dr. Kristal wants to share his knowledge with all of us. All those who wish to be as healthy as they can be, and especially those with health problems that defy conventional treatments, should read this book. I recommend it most highly.

—JOHN R. LEE, M.D.

John R. Lee, M.D. is an internationally recognized authority on women's health and the use of natural hormone replacement therapy. He is the author of several best-selling books, including What Your Doctor May Not Tell You about Menopause, What Your Doctor May Not Tell You about Premenopause, *and* What Your Doctor May Not Tell You about Breast Cancer.

Preface

The Road to Health Is Paved with Misconceptions

Most health-conscious people are aware of the necessity to eat good food and take supplements. People are health-conscious because they desire a continued or better state of health: more energy, restful sleep, and freedom from the many diseases and subclinical syndromes that plague us. Quality of health and life are the hallmarks of most health-conscious individuals. However, the stumbling blocks are many, as most people do not understand their own particular dietary or supplementary needs. The last book or article that a person reads is usually their guideline. It might advise eating for your blood type, vegetarianism, a high protein and high fat diet, a low-fat diet, raw foods, even raw meat—the list goes on and on, and so does the confusion. When I lecture to the lay public, the most common concern I hear is over the conflicting advice from various authorities about what is the most appropriate diet. The confusion stems from the simple fact that *there is no one perfect diet for everyone*. What might be optimal for one person may be the nemesis of another. Just as the road to hell is paved with good intentions, so too is the road to health paved with misconceptions.

To smooth out the bumps on the road to health, and to bring some clarity to this ongoing saga, we might review the historical data. However, the enormous contribution of the great nutritionists of the past would fill a huge number of volumes. Each imparts his or her own understanding and expertise for the enhancement of health. Why then is this pyramiding of knowledge so confusing to the average health-conscious person?

There is a lot more that we do *not* know about health and diseases than we *do* know. Herein lies the root of the confusion. So many theories have been advanced with few facts to back them up. If we were mechanical enti-ties, then one diet might indeed be appropriate for all. But, as we are each biological entities with our own complex biochemical makeup, foods and supplements affect us differently. This is the basis for the revolutionary the-ories of Metabolic Typing, or Personalized Metabolic Nutrition. There are four basic Metabolic Types that we will be exploring in this book (Fast Oxi-dizer, Slow Oxidizer, Sympathetic, and Parasympathetic) but there are many differing gradations within each type.

Personalized Metabolic Nutrition or Metabolic Typing is a system for discerning your Metabolic Type, a term which essentially refers to the char-acteristic way your body produces and processes energy. Although energy is the universal constant that enlivens all of our bodies, it is processed differently by each of the Metabolic Types. Once your Metabolic Type is determined, you can then determine the optimal fuel, or food, that is best suited for your particular metabolism. Different Metabolic Types require different fuel, and varying qualities within each of the Metabolic Types may suggest further modifications of the basic foods and supplements generally recommended for that type.

Thus we arrive at the understanding that we all require different diets. *The Nutrition Solution* presents a reliable testing procedure for determining an individual's Metabolic Type and nutritional protocol. I do not wish to infer that this represents some kind of finality in our understanding of nutri-tion, but it does offer a revolutionary new way to help people help them-selves. Though the methodology is sophisticated, the testing is fairly easy to perform, either by a trained healthcare practitioner or by yourself at home. Armed with this important information, the road to health need no longer be paved with misconceptions.

—HAROLD J. KRISTAL, D.D.S.

Chapter 1

The Theory of Metabolic Typing

My Nutritional Odyssey

Two events from my younger days stand out as influences on my growing awareness of the importance of nutrition. The first took place during my undergraduate years at the University of Minnesota. During a question-and-answer period, I asked my professor, who was the head of the Pharmacology Department, what he thought about people taking vitamins and minerals. His answer was that he thought nutritional supplements would not hurt anyone, and, if they felt better taking them, he had no objection. However, in his opinion, they did not really help to keep people healthy. Now, fifty years later, I ponder the degree to which the mainstream medical community still tends to cling to this same limited understanding.

The second event that took place in my early days was a chance meeting with the author Adelle Davis, one of the first writers to popularize the use of whole foods and nutritional supplements. She had been invited to be a guest speaker at one of our Dental Medicine Seminars in Palm Springs, California, where she enthusiastically espoused the virtues of vitamin C as a preventative for everything from the common cold to cancer. Unfortunately, our esteemed group deemed this point of view to be heretical, dismissing it out of hand as non-scientific quackery, so they unceremoniously ushered her off the podium and would not let her continue her lecture!

But a small group of us thought otherwise, and we invited Ms. Davis to come up to Berkeley to give a one-day seminar. During this time she discovered that I loved peanut butter. "Dr. Kristal," she said, "if you are going to eat peanut butter, always be sure to eat the kind with the oil separated out on top. Never eat hydrogenated, processed peanut butter." Now, hydrogenation (which involves the use of extreme heat and heavy metal catalysts) is intended to preserve the oils in peanut butter and so prevent rancidity, or spoilage. However, hydrogenation "preserves" the oils so well—rendering them chemically closer to plastic than to a food substance—that our bodies are unable to properly break them down, and thus these denatured oils—known as *trans* fats, or *trans* fatty acids—become absorbed into our cell membranes where they wreak havoc with normal cellular metabolism, potentially contributing to all manner of degenerative diseases. Adelle Davis warned me about this back in the 1950s, long before the dangers of hydrogenation and *trans* fats were well known. I feel that she might have quite literally saved my life, as I have consumed untold gallons of this wonderful food since then! As soon as the organic form of peanut butter became available, I began using it exclusively. To this day I have the greatest respect and admiration for Adelle Davis who, perhaps more than any other single individual, ignited my passion for nutrition, as well as that of millions of her readers.

Peanuts share with grapes the dubious distinction of being one of the most heavily sprayed of all commercial food crops. Grapes feature in another incident that occurred several years ago that gave me first-hand experience of the importance of eating organically grown foods. The bunch of Thompson seedless grapes that I purchased from the corner supermarket looked so delicious and fresh. That evening I rinsed them and ate a generous portion; but, later that night and into the early morning hours, I had a severe sinus attack. The cause was completely unknown to me at the time, so the following evening I again happily consumed a quantity of grapes from the same bunch, only to experience the same discomfort as the night before.

By this time I was starting to suspect that the grapes might be responsible. Later the next day I went to a natural food store and purchased some organic grapes. I again ate a similar quantity, but this time I experienced no discomfort whatsoever. To make certain that the original grapes were indeed the culprit, I decided to re-test them and eat them again the next evening. Sure enough, I experienced the same discomfort and congestion as I had on the two previous occasions. This taught me a major lesson about the importance of eating organically grown foods whenever possible. How many of us suffer from similar allergic reactions to pesticides, herbicides, and other contaminants in our foods, without ever suspecting the true cause?

During the last twenty years of my dental practice, I incorporated nutritional consultation more and more into my work. Much of this centered around detoxification protocols for my dental patients before, during, and after the removal of mercury amalgams ("silver" fillings). It is much easier to remove toxic metals from the teeth than from body tissues, which is where they end up after leaching out of the teeth. The substances we used for detoxification included the algae chlorella, cilantro, N-acetyl cysteine (NAC), CoQ10, and antioxidant enzymes (glutathione peroxidase, superoxide dismutase [SOD], catalase, and methionine reductase). I also sometimes suggested intravenous chelation therapy, using DMPS, an effective method for removing ("chelating") mercury from the bloodstream. Today various new oral agents (such as DMSA) also show promise as effective chelators.

My growing understanding of the importance of vitamins and minerals led me to constantly read the emerging literature on the subject. I also took continuing education courses from such notables as Jeffrey Bland, Ph.D., Emmanuel Cheraskin, M.D., Nobel laureate Linus Pauling, Ph.D., and Hans Selye, M.D. who educated the world about the important role played by stress in the development of disease processes. Digesting the wisdom of these great researchers, I became convinced that degenerative diseases were caused primarily by metabolic imbalances, setting the stage for my later discovery of the crucial role of the Metabolic Types. Mercury, for instance, causes numerous disruptions in bodily metabolism, but perhaps the most important is the suppression of the immune system. Mercury (as well as nickel, another commonly used dental material) reduces the quantity of T-lymphocytes (white blood cells), as well qualitatively changing the ratio between the all-important T4 and T8 helper cells. This directly contributes to the development of many degenerative diseases by reducing our immune competence.

My Introduction to the Oxidative System of Metabolic Typing

I was the chairman of the University of California Holistic Study Group from 1983 to 1988. One of my responsibilities as chairman was to provide full-day programs that would enhance our collective knowledge of alternative medical procedures. This was a very exciting time for me, as I had the privilege of choosing and introducing the speakers that I wanted. Some of the notable guests that I brought to speak before the group were John R. Lee, M.D., Richard Kunin, M.D., Edward Winger, M.D., Parris Kidd, Ph.D., Marcel Vogel, Phylis Saifer, M.D., Michael Rosenbaum, M.D., and Jeffrey Bland, Ph.D.

Most of our meetings were held at the university in the medical post-graduate division. However, the university administration was not in alignment with our thinking on such subjects as acupuncture, homeopathy, nutrition, and the toxicity of fluoride and mercury, so before each meeting, I had to get permission from the deans of both the Dental and Medical Schools to present the program. Because they were unwilling to allow certain speakers to appear on the university premises, they refused more programs than they accepted! Fortunately I had a fairly large seminar room above my dental office in Point Richmond, so in the mid 1980s I decided to move the meetings there.

Our meetings were very stimulating and educational, and we all benefited from being exposed to this newfound knowledge. After one of these meetings, while I was cleaning up and rearranging the chairs, I noticed a book left behind on the floor. I picked it up to see if I could find out to whom it belonged, but there was nothing to identify the owner. It turned out to be a book by George Watson, Ph.D., titled *Nutrition and Your Mind: The Psychochemical Response.* I started thumbing through it, and found that I could not put it down. I ended up reading the entire book late into the night!

This book literally changed my life, as it opened up to me the new world of blood pH. Watson had developed a protocol for assessing the health of individuals suffering from what appeared to be mental imbalances, based on the acidity or alkalinity of their venous blood. He described a process known as the Krebs cycle in a way I had not previously understood, emphasizing the varying speeds at which the mitochondria—or "energy furnaces" found in almost all of the cells of the body—convert the nutrients extracted from our food into energy. He based his treatment protocols on how quickly or slowly the individual metabolized (or "oxidized") the nutrients in their foods. Using this radical approach, which centered around diet and nutritional supplementation, he had great success in treating people who were supposedly suffering from psychological imbalances. Though this did not gain him too many friends in the psychoanalytic community, he went on to become a full professor of Philosophy of Science at the University of Southern California. Rudolf

Wiley, Ph.D. later extended Watson's work, and described it in detail in his own book, *BioBalance.*

Initially, I used the same intravenous blood pH testing procedure that Rudolf Wiley used, and tested over three hundred patients with this method. However, this procedure is quite time-consuming, impractical, and invasive, requiring four blood samples to be drawn from a vein in the arm over a fourteen-hour period, while the patient is put on a special restricted diet. I decided to simplify the protocol, relying instead on small amounts of capillary blood taken from a finger stick at timed intervals over a two-hour period, during a modified glucose challenge. I was very successful with this procedure and was able to obtain similar results to those of Watson and Wiley.

My Introduction to the Integrated System of Metabolic Typing

In January 1996 I published an article about my work, titled "The Confusion of Vegetarianism," in the *Townsend Letter for Doctors,* a leading journal for alternative health practitioners. Among the flood of calls I received in response to the article was one from a nutritionist named William (Bill) Wolcott. He was very excited about the article, but insisted that I was only seeing part of the metabolic picture. He explained that only half of the population derive their energy oxidatively (i.e. by converting nutrients into energy via the Krebs cycle), and that the other half derive it autonomically (via the neuro-hormonal system, under the control of the autonomic nervous system). He cited the work of Francis M. Pottenger, M.D. and his own mentor William Donald Kelley, D.D.S. to substantiate this claim. Furthermore, he asserted that *the very same foods and supplements would have opposite pH effects in the Oxidative Metabolic Types as they would in the Autonomic Metabolic Types.* He explained his theory of metabolic dominance: that *either* the Oxidative system *or* the Autonomic system is more active, or dominant, in any given individual; and that, although we all have both systems operating in us, one predominates over the other. Thus an individual would be seen as *either* an Oxidative *or* an Autonomic type. The pH of the blood could then be used to determine which sub-type within the dominant metabolic system characterized the individual. Individuals who operated primarily under the influence of the Oxidative system would be typed as Fast Oxidizers if they had acid blood, or Slow Oxidizers if they had alkaline blood. If, however, they primarily operated under the influence of the Autonomic system, they would be typed as Sympathetics if they had acid blood, or Parasympathetics if they had alkaline blood.

I was so immersed in Watson's Oxidative protocol at the time that I was not very open to Wolcott's suggestions; but his parting remark to me was that if any of my clients did not respond to the Oxidative approach, to try viewing and treating them through the Autonomic system. The very next day, a female patient arrived at my office whose blood test showed her to be overly alkaline. I therefore determined her to be a Slow Oxidizer (the only alkaline blood type in the Oxidative System) and put her on what should have been the appropriate diet for her type. To my amazement she returned the following week feeling worse than before! When I re-tested her blood, I found that it had become even *more* alkaline than it had been when I first saw her, rather than more acid as I had expected and hoped that it would become. I immediately recalled my conversation with Bill Wolcott, and his claim that Autonomic types respond the opposite way as the Oxidative types to the very same foods and supplements.

So, as an experiment, I decided to put her on the opposite kind of diet (a diet that would be expected to further alkalize an Oxidative type), and she returned a couple of weeks later feeling great. When I checked her blood, it had become more acid, something that could not be explained within the Oxidative model, but that could be explained within the Autonomic model. The alkaline blood type in the Autonomic system (the Parasympathetic) requires the totally opposite kind of diet to acidify and, therefore, balance him or her as does the Oxidative alkaline type (the Slow Oxidizer). I excitedly called Bill Wolcott, and so began an intensive three-year conversation that led, through numerous revisions, to the prototype of the current testing and analysis protocols of Metabolic Typing. It is the distillation of this in-depth dialogue between us—explored through extensive telephone, e-mail, and fax communications—that we will be exploring in this book.

The material I am writing about is not widely known in the mainstream medical community, but it does represent a big breakthrough in furthering our understanding of the foods and supplements that work best for people of different Metabolic Types. My work revolves around using different foods to balance the pH of the blood, which in turn leads to an upgrading or optimizing of all the metabolic systems of the body. The big practical distinction between the Oxidative and Autonomic Systems is that *foods that acidify members of one group will alkalize members of the other group, and vice versa.* What I refer to throughout this book as Group I foods (foods lower in protein and fat, and higher in complex carbohydrates) acidify the blood of the Oxidative dominant types, but alkalize the blood of the Autonomic dominant types. Conversely, Group II foods (higher in protein and fat, and lower in carbohydrates) alkalize the blood of the Oxidative dominant types, but acidify the blood of the Autonomic dominant types. In other words, *the same foods produce opposite effects in members of the two different dominance systems,* the Oxidative and the Autonomic (see Figure 1-1).

Bill Wolcott and I decided to design a clinical study to objectively verify our empirical observation that the same foods had different pH effects on the two dominance systems. We enlisted the help of Gabriel Cousens, M.D., who tested a group of eight individuals, using both the modified glucose challenge protocol that I had pioneered and venous blood plasma drawn from the arm. The venous plasma test was administered following the ingestion of fruit and vegetable juices, as well as following the ingestion of a protein powder. The results, which I presented to the annual meeting of the Orthomolecular Health-Medicine Society in San Francisco in March 1998, clearly demonstrated that our hypothesis was correct. The fruit and vegetable juices (representing the Group I foods) had an acidifying effect on the blood pH of the Oxidative dominant types, but an alkalizing effect on the Autonomic dominant types; while the protein powder (representing the Group II foods) had an alkalizing effect on the Oxidative types, but an acidifying effect on the Autonomic

Metabolic Dominance Systems

FIGURE 1-1

Oxidative System
(the conversion of food to energy)

Autonomic System
(neuroendocrine control of energy)

Slow Oxidizers
Alkaline Blood
Group I foods acidify their blood, which balances their blood pH

Fast Oxidizers
Acid Blood
Group II foods alkalize their blood, which balances their blood pH

Sympathetics
Acid Blood
Group I foods alkalize their blood, which balances their blood pH

Parasympathetics
Alkaline Blood
Group II foods acidify their blood, which balances their blood pH

BLOOD PH

It should be noted that, in our discussion of blood pH, we are using the terms *acid* and *alkaline* in a very specific and relative sense. In actuality, all blood is alkaline, as human life could not be supported if it were literally acid. However, blood is alkaline to varying degrees. The pH scale—which measures degrees of acidity and alkalinity—runs from zero (which is extremely acid) to 14 (which is extremely alkaline), with the midpoint of 7 representing the neutral position. Although there is some disagreement about the exact number, I follow George Watson in believing that the ideal venous blood pH is 7.46, which is mildly alkaline. The body strives very hard to maintain the blood pH as close to

this ideal as possible, and it never varies much more than two tenths of a percent on either side of the ideal. There are, however, significant metabolic implications to even these small variations. When we use the term *acid*, we simply mean that the person's blood is showing a tendency to dip below the ideal position of 7.46 (perhaps as low as 7.25), and is therefore on the acid side of the ideal, closer to the acid end of the spectrum; but technically it is still alkaline, albeit weakly so. Conversely, when we use the term *alkaline*, we mean a blood pH that is tending to rise above the ideal of 7.46 (perhaps as high as 7.65), and is, therefore, overly alkaline (see Figure 1-2). All blood is alkaline in the absolute sense; it is simply a matter of degree. For the sake of convenience, we will be using the terms acid and alkaline to signify these degrees.

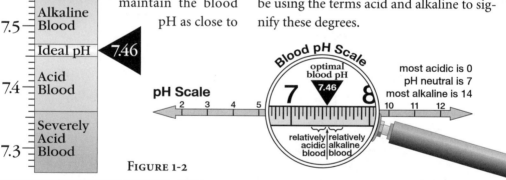

FIGURE 1-2

types.[1] At this time, more is known about how the Oxidative system produces its pH effects than the Autonomic system. Hopefully, in the near future, further research will allow us to better understand why the Autonomic system produces different pH responses to food than the Oxidative system.

In the pages that follow, I will be presenting an overview of the procedures we use in our office to metabolically type our clients. I will also explore in depth the *Personalized Metabolic Nutrition Self-Test,* developed for individuals to use in the comfort and convenience of their own homes. I will also present a simplified questionnaire for immediate use, so that readers will have all the information they need to decide how to best take advantage of this methodology. (A step-by-step *Practitioners' Manual* detailing all the testing protocols, as well as full instructions on how to analyze the data, is available to healthcare practitioners who participate in *Personalized Metabolic Nutrition Seminars.*)

The term *biochemical individuality* was coined by the great biochemist Dr. Roger Williams to indicate the infinite variations in our metabolic biochemistry.[2] Biochemical individuality implies that different ratios of macronutrients (protein, fats, and carbohydrates) and micronutrients (vitamins and minerals) are required for each of us. Yet there are many authors advocating only one type of diet for everyone: Dean Ornish, M.D. recommends a low protein, low fat, high carbohydrate diet;[3] Robert Atkins, M.D. recommends a high protein, high fat, low carbohydrate diet;[4] Barry Sears, Ph.D. weighs in with his Zone Diet, consisting of 40% carbohydrates, 30% proteins, and 30% fats;[5] and so on. If it is true, as Dr. Williams has so elegantly asserted, that our metabolic biochemistry has infinite variations, then *there can be no one diet that is appropriate for everyone.* As the old saying goes, one man's food is another man's poison. Or, in popular parlance, "different strokes for different folks." Our work with Metabolic Typing has confirmed that while there are some foods that are bad for everyone (such as refined sugar, processed foods, and partially hydrogenated oils), *there are also good foods that are bad for you, and good foods that are good for you.* This is determined by your Metabolic Type, which can be understood to be the particular "style" by which your body produces and processes energy.

Venous blood pH is considered ideal at 7.46, because that is the pH at which nutrients can be optimally assimilated and utilized. When you know your Metabolic Type, foods and supplements for your particular profile should bring you nearer to the ideal pH. Being able to utilize macro- and micronutrients optimally will promote a heightened degree of well-being. Energy will tend to be enhanced, allergies will often diminish or disappear, and various disease processes may be slowed or even reversed. In this way

Metabolic Typing is able to offer a much more reliable success rate than more conventional nutritional approaches.

The Jason Kristal Story: U.S. Junior Super Heavyweight Weightlifting Champion

I fathered three children during my first marriage—Sharon, Alan, and Cary. Sharon went on to become a CPA; Alan graduated from the University of Minnesota as a cultural anthropologist, and now works as a specialist in the computer field; but Cary tragically lost his life at the age of nineteen in Mexico. During my second marriage, I fathered two more children, Jason and Allison. Jason, who is now twenty-two, is finishing his college training in law enforcement. Allison, a straight-A student, entered the University of California at Santa Barbara when she was only sixteen years old, and graduated at the age of twenty. Even through I will be dwelling on Jason's achievements, I wish to state emphatically that I am very proud of all my children and their many accomplishments.

I would like to tell you about Jason, and how Metabolic Typing contributed to his success. For four years in a row (from 1996 to 1999), Jason was the National Super Heavyweight Weightlifting Champion in the Junior Division (twenty years old, or younger), breaking national records in all categories. At age sixteen, he won his first gold medal in the national weightlifting championships, and broke the world record in the dead-lift at the California State Powerlifting Championship. At age nineteen, he broke the U.S. heavyweight records in all categories, and was a resident athlete at the Olympic Village in Colorado Springs, Colorado. During his residency, he competed for the United States in his division around the world, as well as here at home. I was present when the International Junior Olympic Event was held in Savannah, Georgia in July of 2000, with approximately one thousand world-class junior weightlifters present from around the world. It was at this event that Jason broke the United States super heavyweight record for juniors, and went on to bring the U.S. its first bronze medal in the junior super heavyweight division.

At just shy of six feet three inches tall, his weight at that time was 310 pounds, with 15% body fat. Upon arriving back at the Olympic Village after his wonderful showing at the international event in Savannah, the Olympic

Committee approached him and told him he could be the Super Heavyweight Champion of the world, but he would need to gain another fifty or sixty pounds. Jason has always been an all-round athlete, outstanding in several sports, such as tennis, football, baseball, and water polo. The idea of gaining the additional weight did not sit well with him, so he asked for my opinion. These are the exact words I told him: "Gaining the extra weight will definitely shorten your life expectancy, and you cannot expect to be as healthy; but if the glory of being world champion is more important to you, you should go for it." In two days, he packed his bags and headed home, resigning his Olympic residency. He chose health over glory. At the time of this writing, Jason weighs in at 235 pounds, with less than 10% body fat, and he still works out three to five hours a day because he enjoys it so much. Jason recently graduated from the San Francisco Police Academy, and is now working as a police officer for the SFPD while finishing his last year in college, where he will receive his B.S. degree in Criminal Justice.

Metabolically, Jason is a Fast Oxidizer. He bases his diet around Group II foods and takes Group II supplements (see Chapter 3 for more information on these protocols). I worked very closely with him during his competitive days, and gave him additional supplements—such as glucosamine and chondroitin sulfate, and MSM—to take care of his aching muscles and joints after

FIGURE 1-3

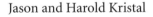

Jason and Harold Kristal

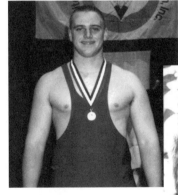

Jason Kristal at
an international
Olympic event

strenuous workouts. We beefed up his amino acid intake to give him greater endurance and strength—using creatine, arginine, ornithine, glutamine, and lysine—and he told me that the amino acids helped him considerably. Jason never drank alcohol, smoked cigarettes, or took drugs, and he scrupulously avoided taking steroids, despite their widespread popularity among weightlifters. He was completely focused on being the very best he could be. His dedication and tenacity were wonderful for me to behold, and I am proud to say I fathered one of the strongest athletes in the United States for four years in a row. I am very proud of Jason's accomplishments, as well as his decision to remain healthy.

I myself have played singles' tennis almost every day for the last thirty-one years. I felt that running around the tennis court every day for an hour and a half was all the exercise I needed; but Jason convinced me to work out at Gold's Gym with him. He put me on a seventy-minute body-building program which has given me a huge boost, both mentally and physically. My chronological age is seventy-seven, but my biological age is probably closer to fifty. My exercise program today consists of sixty minutes of singles' tennis and seventy minutes of body-building exercises, seven days a week if my schedule permits it.

The Trilogy of Health

There are three primary aspects to good health, which we can refer to as a *trilogy of health*. Each one is essential to maintain the proper balance of factors that defines good health. Although the focus of this book is on the third member of this trilogy—nutrition—I would be remiss if I did not mention all three.

The Trilogy of Health
Mental Attitude
Exercise
Diet and Nutrition

What *is* mental attitude? It can be understood as the mental stance we take toward life based on the sum total of our past experiences. These experiences have molded our character, attitudes, and thoughts. Even though we live in the here-and-now, the ground of our mental attitude has been fertilized by the experiences of the past. Some of these have been painful and traumatic, while others have been uplifting and inspiring. It is not necessarily the balance between these types of experience that colors our attitude toward life, but rather how we perceive them. Our perceptions and beliefs essentially shape the reality of life in the here-and-now. My own belief is that life is precious. We are on this beautiful earth for a very short time, and so my choice is to be as happy and healthy as I possibly can. Love of humanity, love of oneself, and whole-hearted engagement in whatever endeavor one pursues is my blueprint for a happy and productive life. One's mental attitude can always be changed for the positive, both for the betterment of oneself and the world around us.

Exercise is very important to one's overall sense of well-being because it stimulates and vitalizes all the organs, glands, and tissues of our body. Not only does it strengthen the muscles and the heart, but it also oxygenates the brain. In this way, exercise can help to keep us mentally sharp, while also increasing the production of the feel-good neurotransmitters, brain chemicals that play a key role in determining mood. Successful weight loss is often not possible without exercise. Trying to lose weight through nutritional means alone is like fighting with one hand tied behind your back. While the right diet may be the most important factor in weight loss, it is greatly assisted by a complementary exercise program tailored to the needs and capacities of the individual.

Physical exercise and athletic capacity have been respected for centuries throughout the world, and are perhaps best exemplified by the Olympic Games. We cannot all be Olympians, nor do we need to be in order to maintain good health, but we can all embrace an exercise program to mobilize the one hundred trillion cells in our body. Each person needs to find a form of exercise that both suits their temperament and their physical capabilities— whether it is competitive sports, running, bicycling, swimming, working out at the gym, practicing yoga or a martial art, or simply walking around their neighborhood. Walking is a very underestimated form of exercise, partly because it lacks the glamour of other activities, and partly because it appears to require less exertion. Nevertheless, it promotes good circulation, muscle and bone strength, and flexibility, while helping to regulate blood sugar levels, stimulate hormone production, and oxygenate the brain. It is also a great way to de-stress after a hectic day at work, while reconnecting with one's environment; literally and figuratively it provides a simple way to stop and smell the roses. Many great thinkers (from the poet William Wordsworth to the Nobel prize winning physicist Nils Bohr) received much of their inspiration during their daily walks. As an added bonus, it requires no special equipment (except a good pair of shoes), costs nothing, can be done anywhere, alone or with a companion, and by almost anyone.

Dr. Carl Simonton, author of the book *Getting Well Again,* always put his cancer patients on some sort of physical exercise program, ranging from calisthenics to walking.[6] I once had the opportunity to debate Covert Bailey, a well-known lecturer on physical fitness, on whether exercise is more important than diet, or vice versa. I took the position that diet is more important, though I have come to believe that both are vital to good health. Neither one of us convinced the other, but we did end up agreeing on the value of both.

Nutrition also has the ability to affect changes in mental attitude, as the health of the hundred trillion cells in our body is directly affected by diet. The micronutrients that are required by our brain cells for proper neurotransmitter activity come from our food; so if we feed our body poor quality food, or if our digestive system is under-performing, the very functioning of the brain can be compromised. Not only must we eliminate foods that are bad for everyone (such as sugar, white flour, and refined oils), but we must also eat for our Metabolic Type. The best food for any given individual can be determined through the testing protocols of Metabolic Typing. Optimizing health through sound nutrition—as well as by cultivating a positive mental attitude, and finding a suitable exercise program— should be a goal shared by everyone.

ALLOPATHIC NUTRITION VERSUS METABOLIC NUTRITION
~

Modern medicine has made great strides in developing sophisticated diagnostic technology, and is very proficient at handling acute and emergency care. However, it is poorly equipped to combat chronic disease, and even less successful in addressing the almost universal desire of individuals to simply *feel better:* to have more energy, and to have it be more consistent throughout the day; to be more resistant to the negative effects of stress; and to be more capable of fending off illness, whether it be the common cold or the so-called diseases of aging. This is where Metabolic Typing comes in. Whereas modern medicine is, first and foremost, a disease-care system, Metabolic Typing is a true healthcare system. It addresses the individual at a fundamental metabolic level, seeking to optimize whole body health and well-being. Knowing one's Metabolic Type—the fundamental way in which the body produces and processes energy—an individual can knowingly select the foods and nutritional supplements that are tailored to his or her specific metabolism.

However, most nutritionists today practice what I call *allopathic nutrition;* that is, utilizing a specific nutrient or nutritional protocol as a universal treatment for a given condition. For example: calcium is generally recommended to individuals with osteoporosis; niacin for high cholesterol or poor circulation; and vitamin B-6 for circulatory disorders. These various supplements are often advocated to treat their respective disorders irrespective of the unique qualities that make up each individual's metabolism. This is the essence of the allopathic approach to nutrition. What is so confusing and confounding about nutrition today is that some people are helped by these protocols while others are not. Some, perhaps, are even made worse. The late Roger J. Williams, Ph.D., noted biochemist from the University of Texas, coined the term *biochemical individuality* to indicate that we are all biochemically unique. We now understand that these biochemical differences define an individual's Metabolic Type. My experience has led me to believe that, when it comes to nutrition, it is the difference between Metabolic Types that accounts for the observation that what makes one person better may do absolutely nothing for someone else with the same condition, or may possibly even make them worse.

Premises of Metabolic Typing

1. *Metabolism* can be defined as the sum total of all life-supporting biochemical and electrical reactions that take place in a cell or organism.

2. *Metabolism* is regulated by a number of homeostatic control mechanisms, physiological processes that work to maintain a dynamic equilibrium (or homeostasis) in the body.

3. *Ideal venous blood pH of 7.46* reflects the biochemical balance and metabolic efficiency of the homeostatic control mechanisms. Anything below a blood pH of 7.46 is overly acid; anything above is overly alkaline. If the blood pH is at the ideal level, then optimum absorption and utilization of micro- and macronutrients will take place. The further the pH deviates from the ideal, the less efficient will be the absorption and utilization of these nutrients. This creates an imbalanced milieu in which allergies, fatigue, digestive disorders, and a multitude of other disease conditions can occur.

4. *The two most fundamental homeostatic control mechanisms* that regulate blood pH are the rate of oxidation (or energy production) and the action of the autonomic nervous system.

5. *The Oxidative types* are defined by the oxidation rate, the speed at which the conversion of nutrients into energy occurs intracellularly (within the cells of the body). Two sub-types are defined by the oxidation rate: the Fast Oxidizer (who produces an acid deviation in blood pH); and the Slow Oxidizer (who produces an alkaline deviation in blood pH); either of these two sub-types would be considered a Balanced Oxidizer when they produce a balanced blood pH.

6. *The Autonomic types* are defined by the relative dominance of the two divisions of the autonomic (or involuntary) nervous system (ANS), the master regulator of metabolism. Two sub-types are defined by the ANS: the Sympathetic type (who produces an acid deviation in blood pH); and the Parasympathetic type (who produces an alkaline deviation in blood pH); either of these two sub-types would be considered a Balanced Autonomic type when they produce a balanced blood pH.

7. *Overly acid or alkaline blood pH* can be due *either* to the influence of the Oxidative system *or* the Autonomic system. *The most significant difference between these two systems is that most foods and most nutrients that acidify the Oxidative types alkalize the Autonomic types, and foods and nutrients that alkalize the Oxidative types acidify the Autonomic types.*

The Dominance Factor

The importance of the dominance factor was first observed and formulated by William L. Wolcott in 1983. He realized that the effect of any food or nutrient on an individual's biochemistry is not solely the result of the inherent (or absolute) qualities of the substance itself, but rather of the influence of the control system (either the Oxidative or the Autonomic) that is dominant in controlling the person's metabolism. This explains why a given nutrient can have such different effects in different people. It also explains why what works for one person with a given condition may not work for another person with the same condition.

When health practitioners use nutrition to address disease states without taking into consideration their Metabolic Type, they are employing an allopathic approach. This is because any given nutrient can be either acidifying *or* alkalizing, depending upon one's Metabolic Type. Whether the protocol is right or wrong will depend on whether or not the recommendations are suitable for the individual's Metabolic Type. Otherwise the success or failure of the treatment will be hit-or-miss, a matter of chance, not predictability.

Keep in mind that foods and supplements will be either acid or alkaline forming in the body, depending upon the dominant control system. For example, calcium—which is currently universally recommended for bone loss—is alkaline forming for the Oxidative types and acid forming for the Autonomic types. Fast Oxidizers with bone loss will benefit from calcium because it will help to alkalize them. However, Slow Oxidizers are already too alkaline, and will therefore be further alkalized by calcium; they need to limit their calcium intake and, instead, increase potassium, magnesium, and manganese (which are acid forming in the Oxidative system) to improve the utilization of the calcium which they already have. Conversely, calcium is acid forming for the Autonomic types. Therefore, taking calcium would be desirable for the Parasympathetic, who runs on the overly alkaline side, but not for the Sympathetic, who already is overly acidic. The Sympathetic, like the Slow Oxidizer, should instead emphasize potassium, magnesium, and manganese, which are alkalizing for the Autonomic types.

The metabolic approach to nutrition involves *first* determining the individual's Metabolic Type, and *then* making nutritional recommendations to address the underlying imbalance in the fundamental homeostatic mechanism. On the basis of this understanding, I believe that it is no longer sufficient to approach nutrition allopathically. One must first understand the individual's Metabolic Type, and then proceed metabolically.

When a person is balanced metabolically, many disease symptoms subside. These can include chronic conditions with no previously observable cause. Allergies that a person might have had for years might disappear; fatigue problems may be alleviated; and digestive disorders often resolve. This is because the body is now able to utilize nutrients optimally. However, it is important to understand that *in none of these instances is the condition itself being directly treated. Rather, it is the imbalance in the underlying homeostatic control mechanism that is being addressed.*

The Forerunners: Pottenger, Watson, and Kelley

The foundation for Metabolic Typing was laid by several great scientists. It is difficult to do justice to the monumental contributions Francis M. Pottenger, M.D., George Watson, Ph.D., and William Donald Kelley, D.D.S. have made to the fields of health, nutrition, and medicine. The combined results of their foresight and pioneering research prepared the groundwork for an evolving new nutritional analysis and clinical system which holds out the promise of changing the way nutrition and, potentially, medicine itself will be practiced in the future.

The name Francis M. Pottenger, M.D. is most often associated with the famous Pottenger Cat Studies, which were actually performed by his son, Francis M. Pottenger Jr., M.D., in the 1930s and 1940s.[7] Indeed, this line of research was most valuable in illuminating the influences of certain nutrients, or the lack thereof, on the processes of growth, reproduction, and degenerative conditions. Of equal importance, though not as widely known, was the senior Pottenger's study of the relationship of nutrition to the sympathetic and parasympathetic divisions of the autonomic nervous system, which he carefully delineated in *Symptoms of Visceral Disease.*[8]

The autonomic nervous system (ANS) is the part of the nervous system that generally operates outside our conscious control. The word autonomic, which is essentially synonymous with the word automatic, indicates that the action of the ANS is involuntary, operating below the threshold of our awareness. This distinguishes it from the central nervous system, over which we have direct conscious control. The autonomic nervous system regulates all the vital, moment-to-moment physiological processes that keep the body alive: it keeps the lungs breathing and the blood circulating; it digests and assimilates our food, and eliminates wastes; it distributes the energy produced in the cells of the body; and it regulates the activity of the endocrine glands, such as the thyroid, the adrenals, and the pituitary.

The ANS has two branches or divisions: the sympathetic and the parasympathetic. The sympathetic is the more dynamic or *hyper* branch, and is the part that initiates the famous "flight-or-flight" stress response—stimulating the release of adrenaline, speeding up the heartbeat, and raising the blood pressure. The parasympathetic branch, by contrast, is more *hypo,* concerned with relaxation and digestion ("rest and digest"); it is characterized by a slowing of the heart rate and lowering of the blood pressure. Dr. Pottenger illuminated how the autonomic influences are essential components in defining metabolic individuality. He showed how the action of one branch *or* the other (the sympathetic *or* the parasympathetic) will tend to be predominant in any given individual, and he went on to show how various nutrients activate or inhibit each branch of the ANS. For the two Autonomic types (Sympathetics and Parasympathetics) in whom the ANS is the central influence controlling their metabolism, the goal of our nutritional protocols is to balance its two branches—triggering the underactive branch, and toning down the overactive one. This process is analogous to balancing the two sides of a seesaw. We have extrapolated many of the findings from Pottenger's groundbreaking and reproducible research, and built them into our Metabolic Typing protocol. Dr. Francis M. Pottenger is truly the father of the autonomic (or neuroendocrine) aspect of Metabolic Typing.

George Watson, Ph.D. was a full professor at the University of Southern California. His biochemical research—which spanned the 1950s to the mid-1980s—focused on the role of oxidation in defining metabolic individuality, particularly as it related to psychochemical states and personality disorders. The oxidation rate, as he described it, is the rate of the intracellular conversion of nutrients into energy, involving a chain of biochemical processes that includes glycolysis, the Krebs (or citric acid) cycle, beta-oxidation, and oxidative phosphorylation—collectively leading to the production of energy in the form of ATP. Through objective testing protocols, he classified people as either Fast, Slow, or Sub-Oxidizers.[9] Fast Oxidizers produce an acid venous blood pH, Slow Oxidizers produce an alkaline venous blood pH, while Sub-Oxidizers produce a relatively balanced blood pH. He found that manifestations of physical and psychological imbalance occurred when the venous pH deviated too far from the optimal pH of 7.46. His classic book, *Nutrition and Your Mind,* eloquently describes his fascinating research, and the turnaround that he was able to effect in many of his patients was phenomenal. Rudolf Wiley, Ph.D, later expanded on Watson's work, outlining in his own book, *BioBalance*, a testing methodology that he himself developed.[10] I myself practiced nutrition based upon Watson and Wiley's approach for many years, and I subsequently developed a modified glucose tolerance test to help determine the acid-alkaline balance of the blood, and its relationship to the oxidative processes, from information found in Watson's work.[11] Dr. Watson's oxidative research is of equal importance to Dr. Pottenger's neurohormonal research in laying the groundwork for Metabolic Typing.

William Donald Kelley, D.D.S. has a special place in the hearts of many of his patients who are alive today because of the effectiveness of his unique metabolic protocols. Realizing the deep import of the age-old adage that "one person's food is another person's poison," Kelley was the first to utilize computer technology to analyze the components that comprise metabolic individuality. Basing his work upon Pottenger's original research earlier in the twentieth century, Kelley developed a systematic, testable, and repeatable means of determining Metabolic Type, based exclusively on the autonomic nervous system.[12] Kelley is not currently recognized in traditional medical circles, although he truly deserves such recognition. However, one of his students, Nicholas Gonzalez, M.D., is currently enjoying critical acclaim for his clinical trials with cancer patients, following Kelley's protocols.[13] One of Kelley's patients, who later became a client of mine, was diagnosed with leukemia in 1972. She was advised to have chemotherapy but sought alternative treatment instead. She saw Dr. Kelley in 1972 and underwent a complete remission.

Why is the legacy of these three scientists so important? Separately, each of them broke through the limitations of the research current in their times to make a unique discovery; but, taken together, their collective discoveries give us a fuller sense of the complexities of the human metabolic system. Their work provides the cornerstones of our research in Metabolic Typing, though it took Bill Wolcott's insight and intuition to synthesize all of their work together into one integrated system.

To determine an individual's Metabolic Type, we have developed a simple, accurate methodology utilizing the modified glucose tolerance test, various other objective indicators, and a questionnaire that deals with dietary, physical, and psychological characteristics. From these data we can provide customized dietary and nutritional recommendations, thereby giving concrete answers to the individual's most basic nutritional questions: "What kind of diet should I eat? And what are the specific foods that will sustain and nurture me in good health?" Until now we have had no definitive means of recommending the most appropriate diet, even though it provides the very foundation of our health. Hitherto it has been a matter of trial and error, rather than of science.

Case Histories

As we have seen, there are two primary dominance systems that control human metabolism, the Oxidative and the Autonomic. One *or* the other of these two control systems is understood to be more active in any given individual in regulating their metabolism. Either the Oxidative *or* the Autonomic system will be predominant. Our work is to identify that dominant control system and, further, to determine which of the two sub-types within that system characterizes the individual. If they are an Oxidative type, they will *either* be a Slow *or* Fast Oxidizer; if they are an Autonomic type, they will *either* be a Sympathetic *or* Parasympathetic type. Thus, our strategy in working with clients is first and foremost to address the individual's Metabolic Type, the underlying control mechanism that regulates their particular metabolism. Using nutrition as our tool, we seek to establish homeostasis, or a dynamic equilibrium in the relevant dominance system. If the client is an Oxidative type, we work to modulate their oxidation rate, the rate at which they convert nutrients into energy. With a Slow Oxidizer, we use foods that will speed up their oxidation rate; with a Fast Oxidizer, we use foods that will slow down their oxidation rate. If they are an Autonomic type, we seek to achieve a balance between sympathetic and parasympathetic activity. For a Sympathetic type, we would use targeted nutrition to stimulate the parasympathetic branch; for a Parasympathetic type, we would use nutrients that would help to stimulate the sympathetic branch. The following case histories will help to illustrate this approach.

George is a sixty-seven-year-old man who was slightly overweight, and had elevated cholesterol and triglycerides. His physician had put him on blood pressure medication and suggested a largely vegetarian diet with very little fat. He heard about the work I was doing and scheduled an appointment. For the last several readings his total serum cholesterol had been 216, 219, and 240, while his triglycerides had been mildly elevated at 138, 106, and 115—despite the fact that he was eating a vegetarian diet. I tested him metabolically and found that he was a very Fast Oxidizer. I explained that my focus was to balance his blood pH, and, for his Metabolic Type, this entailed a diet higher in proteins and fats. Although he felt that, together, we were flying in the face of popular belief, he had seen insufficient results thus far with the conventional approach. Three months later George had his next medical test, and his cholesterol was now only 198, and his triglycerides were down to 69 (well into the optimal range of below 100). Additionally, he had lost weight, was more energetic, and his knee problems were somewhat alleviated.

Annie, a lovely fifteen-year-old girl, was brought in by her parents. She was covered with acne pustules all over her body, and also suffered from asthma. For five years, her parents had sought help from both doctors and nutritionists, but to no avail. Through Metabolic Typing, I determined her to be an extremely Fast Oxidizer, with secondary imbalances that included a zinc deficiency. I recommended the appropriate diet and supplements for her Metabolic Type, including essential fatty acids and supplemental zinc. She promised to desist from consuming sugar, and to be diligent with the program. Three weeks later, Annie had improved over 50%. She progressed with each subsequent visit, and after six months she had improved 90–95%. She no longer has asthmatic attacks and does not need an inhaler.

This is an interesting case to further illustrate the difference between the metabolic and allopathic approaches. On the surface, one could say that I had used zinc allopathically, since it is commonly recommended for skin problems. It is also common for zinc supplementation to provide positive results in some cases but not in others; but from a metabolic approach, I knew that additional zinc would be appropriate for a Fast Oxidizer, and would assist in correcting the underlying imbalance. (The deficiency itself likely stemmed from an inability to utilize zinc due to the metabolic imbalance). If she had been a Slow Oxidizer, however, supplemental zinc would have further exacerbated her fundamental imbalance because she would not have been able to metabolize it. In such a case, supplementation with one of the co-factors required for zinc metabolism, rather than zinc itself, would have been more appropriate. Similarly, her particular Metabolic Type requires a greater amount of essential fatty acids than do other types. This same treatment protocol would not have been effective for the same condition in a different Metabolic Type.

A seventy-year-old man named Bill, who was one hundred pounds overweight, visited our office. The testing protocol revealed him to be a Slow Oxidizer, a type that requires a diet low in purine proteins and fats. Although he was already on a vegetarian diet, he was selecting vegetables and legumes that were higher in purines (spinach, artichokes, lentils) and was eating a higher percentage of fats than was right for his type. Adjusting his diet, and supplementing with nutrients supportive to his Metabolic Type, I was able to address the underlying homeostatic imbalance, and he lost seven pounds within the next twenty days.

From an allopathic point of view, one might be tempted to make similar recommendations to all patients desiring to lose weight. But not so from the point of view of Metabolic Typing. A case in point involved John, a seventeen-year-old high school student who was brought in by his parents. He was not very tall, weighed 220 pounds with 50% body fat, and could not compete in athletics. Testing confirmed him to be a Fast Oxidizer. The appropriate protocol for him included a diet high in richer proteins and relatively high in fats, along with specific vegetables and nutrients to support his Metabolic Type. In addition, I recommended supplemental essential fatty acids, digestive enzymes, and an herbal product called *Garcinia cambogia* one half-hour before each meal. One month later, his weight had dropped nineteen pounds (from 220 to 201), and his body fat had dropped 8%, down to 42%. He was feeling much better, and is continuing to lose weight, and is now able to participate in high school athletics.

Additional Case Histories

Another case history involved a fifty-three-year-old woman who suffered from high cholesterol and fatigue. Jean's blood pH was alkaline—which I thought was due to her being a Slow Oxidizer—so I put her on what should have been an acidifying dietary and supplement regime. But when she returned a few weeks later she said she was feeling worse. Upon checking her blood pH, sure enough, she had become even *more* alkaline. (I always recheck clients after approximately four weeks to ensure that we have correctly determined their Metabolic Type). This could *only* mean that she was an Autonomic type, not an Oxidizer as I had initially thought. Had she been a Slow Oxidizer, the foods I had recommended to her (which are acidifying for the Oxidative types) would have acidified her, thereby bringing her more into balance. The fact that these foods actually had the reverse effect and *further* alkalized her meant that she had to be an Autonomic type—because foods that acidify Oxidizers will alkalize Autonomics. Because her blood had become even more alkaline, she therefore had to be a Parasympathetic (the only alkaline Autonomic type). Accordingly, I changed her diet to fit the Parasympathetic profile and, in two weeks, when she reported for follow-up testing, her pH was ideal. She also told me she felt much better and was encouraged by the results. Five weeks later she called back and told me that her fatigue had vanished and her cholesterol had dropped forty points, the lowest it had been in ten years. This kind of balancing of blood cholesterol profiles is frequently seen when a person becomes metabolically balanced.

Another client was a sixty-nine-year-old woman with breast cancer. Gloria had been treated with radiation and chemotherapy following a lumpectomy. Upon being dismissed, she was reassured that the procedure had been successful and that the problem would probably never reoccur. However, one and a half years later, the cancer reappeared, and she was told that she would have to go through the same treatment as before; but she refused to do so, being unwilling to experience the same ordeal all over again. She was then referred to me for nutritional counseling. I informed her that I do not treat cancers, and she should continue to be monitored by her physician, to which she agreed. I discovered that Gloria was a Slow Oxidizer, with extremely alkaline blood. I balanced her pH to near ideal with an acid forming diet appropriate for her Metabolic Type, put her on a strict regime of pancreatic enzymes and selected antioxidants, and checked her every two weeks. After she had been on this nutritional protocol for three months, her energy level had improved and she was not as sickly as she had been. I advised her to have a thorough checkup with her physician, and she was informed by the hospital oncology unit that she had no evidence of any cancer, and was in remission.

CAMILLA'S STORY

Camilla is a sixty-one-year-old woman of Spanish decent who presented with an array of problems: pressure in the left eye from glaucoma, excess weight, lack of energy, a gum infection, stress, and indigestion. She is five feet one inch tall and weighed in at over two hundred pounds, but we were unable to obtain an accurate body fat reading as she exceeded the upper limit of 70% that is detectable by our body fat monitor. She had started putting on excess weight in her mid twenties, after the birth of her daughter. Her diet consisted of the standard American diet (aptly abbreviated to SAD!), with lots of sugar and soft drinks. The primary health complaint that motivated her to seek my services was pressure in the left eye, caused by glaucoma. The only medication she took was aspirin to control the pain in her left eye, and she was not taking any supplements, though she had recently started water aerobics twice a week to help with her weight.

Our test results, which included a strongly acid blood pH reading, indicated a pronounced Group II tendency, requiring a diet higher in protein and fat, and low in carbs. She mentioned that wheat was her favorite grain, and she was regularly consuming a lot of bread and other wheat products. However, electro-dermal testing (performed with an electro-acupuncture device) showed her to be highly allergic to wheat, while also revealing imbalances in 90% of the various organ systems tested. The big question was: would she be willing to give up the wheat products? I also performed a microscopic analysis of her blood, a procedure that I use as a baseline against which I can chart a client's progress. This showed a significant clumping of red blood cells (known as erythrocyte aggregation or rouleau), indicating overly thick (or viscous) blood, along with many misshapen red blood cells (acanthocytes) and considerable cellular dehydration (indicated by target cells or codocytes). This was not a pretty picture! What to do? I was quite confident she was a Fast Oxidizer, one of the two Metabolic Types that typically have a strong negative reaction to wheat; so, I put her on a diet and supplement protocol appropriate for a Fast Oxidizer.

I gave Camilla only six different supplements to take, although there were many additional ones that I could have recommended to her. I have found that it is very difficult for clients to comply if more are recommended, so I decided to give her only the specific ones that I felt would help her the most. Ultimately, the diet is even more important than the supplements. We spent thirty minutes reviewing her dietary and supplement program, to make sure that she felt comfortable with it, and we encouraged her to try to follow it as best she could.

She returned in thirty days beaming. Her first words were that the pressure in her left eye had subsided, and that she had successfully followed the diet and supplement regimen 100%. Her weight had dropped ten pounds, and her body fat now registered at 68.6%. Her blood microscope analysis and electro-dermal testing also improved dramatically, and her blood was 35% less acid. She told me she liked what was happening to her body, but had serious cravings for wheat in the late afternoon. I explained to her that we could help her with these cravings by having her take 1500 mg of the amino acid L-glutamine, two hours after lunch.

I mentioned earlier that Camilla had started to gain weight after the birth of her daughter. There are three issues that I would consider in a case like this one. The first is a possible reproductive hormone imbalance. The second, related, issue has to do with the thyroid gland. It is quite common for the thyroid to reduce its output of the hormone thyroxine as a woman enters her middle years, and the birth of Camilla's daughter may well have accelerated a thyroxine deficiency. Even though childbirth is a natural event, our modern lifestyle tends to complicate it. I suspected that Camilla may well be suffering from sub-clinical hypothyroidism (low thyroid function), and, if she hit a plateau in her weight loss, I might recommend a thyroid glandular product to her. The third issue concerns our vital reserves. We are born with seven times the energy needed to sustain life. How quickly or how slowly we use up these reserves might very well determine the length of our lives, and so preserving these reserves should be our ultimate health goal. People who dissipate their energy will shorten their life span. Camilla had unwittingly been dissipating her reserves over the last thirty-seven years; but, now, with a change in lifestyle, she would be able to preserve and enhance her remaining reserves.

These case histories illustrate how powerful a tool Metabolic Typing can be, and they present a compelling argument for a metabolic, rather than an allopathic approach to nutrition. Treating symptoms alone may succeed sometimes, but addressing the underlying metabolic imbalance is a much more sound and reliable strategy. This is the vision of true healthcare that Metabolic Typing offers to the new millennium, a vision that puts health and well-being front and center, while giving individuals the tools that allow them to take full responsibility for their own health.

MAJOR TENETS OF METABOLIC TYPING

∾ We are all biochemically unique, with different constitutional and genetically inherited nutrient requirements.

∾ People are predisposed to greater or lesser dominance in *either* the Oxidative system (the conversion of nutrients into energy) *or* the Autonomic system (the distribution of that energy via the autonomic nervous system).

∾ The Oxidative system consists of Fast and Slow Oxidizers (determined by the speed at which they convert nutrients into energy).

∾ The Autonomic system consists of Sympathetic and Parasympathetic types (determined by which of the two branches of the autonomic nervous system is more active).

∾ There are foods that are bad for everyone (sugar, white flour products, partially hydrogenated oil, deep-fried foods, chemical additives, etc.).

∾ There are good foods that are bad for you, as well as good foods that are good for you, depending on your Metabolic Type.

∾ Any given nutrient or food can have virtually opposite biochemical effects in individuals of different Metabolic Types.

∾ Foods and nutrients that acidify the two Oxidative types (Fast and Slow Oxidizers) alkalize the two Autonomic types (Sympathetics and Parasympathetics); foods and nutrients that alkalize the Oxidative types, acidify the Autonomic types.

∾ An ideal venous blood pH of 7.46 reflects the biochemical balance and metabolic efficiency of a balanced metabolism.

OXYGEN, CARBON DIOXIDE, AND THE KREBS CYCLE

The Complementary Roles of Oxygen and Carbon Dioxide

We all know that oxygen is absolutely essential to life. We can survive for weeks without food, days without water, but only minutes without oxygen. When tissue levels of oxygen drop too sharply, the brain suffers irreversible damage, the organism can no longer sustain itself, and death occurs. Few of us, however, understand the link between the ordinary act of breathing— or respiration—and the remarkable series of changes that subsequently occur in the lungs, the bloodstream, and the tissues and cells of the body.

As we breathe in, inhaled oxygen (O_2) is absorbed in the walls of the lungs by hemoglobin (a protein-iron component of the red blood cells) and carried off through the bloodstream to tissue cells all over the body, where it performs its vital functions. As we breathe out the process is reversed, only this time it is carbon dioxide (CO_2)—which, like oxygen, is a gas—that is picked up by the hemoglobin molecules and transported away from the tissues to the lungs, to be exhaled (see Figure 1-4). In other words, oxygen is consumed from the outside, but carbon dioxide is produced from within the body. Interestingly, trees and other plants function in reverse from human beings, absorbing or consuming ("breathing in") CO_2 and producing or emitting ("breathing out") oxygen. Thus, our survival needs for oxygen are perfectly complemented by the requirement of plants for CO_2, creating a harmonious symbiosis that is, unfortunately, seriously threatened by the mass destruction of the world's rainforests, which have aptly been described as the lungs of the planet.

Just as we think of oxygen as life-giving, we also tend to think of carbon dioxide as an undesirable waste product. This impression is strengthened by the fact that CO_2 is a common environmental pollutant, associated with heavy industry and acid rain. Released in excessive quantities into the environment, it is indeed very destructive to affected ecosystems. However, in

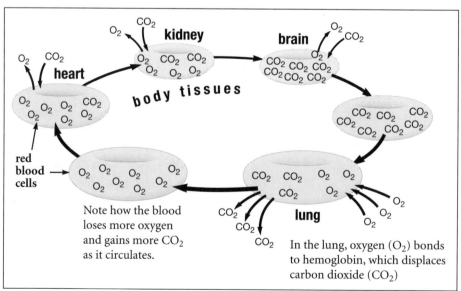

FIGURE 1-4
Oxygen and Carbon Dioxide

Note how the blood loses more oxygen and gains more CO_2 as it circulates.

In the lung, oxygen (O_2) bonds to hemoglobin, which displaces carbon dioxide (CO_2)

THE THEORY OF METABOLIC TYPING 29

the human body, CO_2 performs many vital functions. Foremost among these is its role as the catalyst that allows oxygen to be released from the hemoglobin, freeing it up so that it can be absorbed into the tissue cells of such organs as the kidneys, heart, and brain. In fact, the tissues themselves require approximately three times as much CO_2 as they do oxygen.[14] When the correct ratio exists between these two complementary blood gases, not only is oxygen effectively released into the tissues, but the blood vessels are also more relaxed, edema (the excessive buildup of fluid) is prevented, waste products are more effectively eliminated, and energy production is optimized.

While greater amounts of oxygen may sound desirable, oxygen would remain bound to hemoglobin without sufficient CO_2, leading to oxygen deprivation in the tissues (hypoxia). This is precisely what happens in cases of hyperventilation and panic attacks: too much oxygen is inhaled and too much CO_2 is exhaled. Hence the rationale behind the common practice of breathing into a brown paper bag to recover from hyperventilation; this allows the exhaled CO_2 to be recycled back into the body to correct the imbalance between the two gases.

What does all of this have to do with Metabolic Typing? Oxygen is alkaline forming in the blood, and carbon dioxide acid forming. The optimal ratio between them is intimately connected with maintaining the optimal blood pH of 7.46 which, as we have seen, is the primary goal of Metabolic Typing. At this pH level, all of the systems of the body tend to function harmoniously. If there is an excess of oxygen (or deficit of CO_2) the blood will be overly alkalized. Conversely, if there is an excess of carbon dioxide (or a deficit of oxygen) the blood will be overly acidified (see Figure 1-5). This observation is used during the Metabolic Typing protocol to help determine an individual's Metabolic Type. After taking a series of baseline readings, we administer a glucose challenge drink. This drink is acid forming to the two Oxidative types, thereby increasing their blood levels of CO_2 and decreasing their levels of oxygen. This has the effect of increasing the respiration rate, as the body tries to compensate by breathing in more oxygen, while decreasing the ability to hold the breath, due to a deficit of oxygen. The individuals who demonstrate these traits during the testing procedure (determined by comparing readings taken at a specified time after ingesting the glucose challenge drink with the baseline readings) will generally, therefore, be the Oxidative types. Conversely, the glucose challenge drink is alkalizing to the Autonomic

FIGURE 1-5
Excess Oxygen
and Carbon
Dioxide

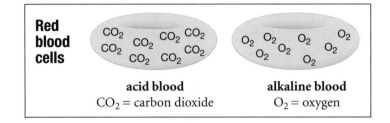

types, thereby increasing blood levels of oxygen and decreasing their levels of CO_2. Accordingly their respiration rate will tend to drop, due to the presence of adequate amounts of oxygen, while their ability to hold their breath will increase. These traits would therefore suggest that an individual demonstrating such a shift is one of the Autonomic types.

The Krebs Cycle

Oxygen and carbon dioxide also play key roles in the production of energy in the Krebs cycle (also known as the citric acid cycle). Inside each of the cells of our body (except mature red blood cells) are hundreds of tiny oval-shaped organelles, microscopic organs known as mitochondria, ranging in number from about 300 in fat cells to 4,000 in heart cells. The mitochondria (or mitochondrion, in the singular) are often referred to as the body's energy furnaces (see Figure 1-6), because it is here that the nutrients extracted from our foods through the digestive process are converted into energy. This happens through a complex set of interactions known as the Krebs cycle (named after its discoverer, Sir Hans Krebs), in association with the electron transport chain which finishes off the work started by the Krebs cycle. While diagrams of the Krebs cycle can look daunting to the layperson (see Figure 1-7), all we need to concern ourselves with here is a basic outline of the biochemical pathways involved.

FIGURE 1-6

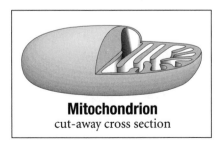

Mitochondrion
cut-away cross section

Essentially, the Krebs cycle involves a series of enzymatic reactions that transform carbohydrates (as glucose, then pyruvate) into intermediate substances. Proteins, in the form of their constituent amino acids, are broken down and fed into the cycle at different points. Fats (as fatty acids) are split into smaller compounds known as ketones or ketone

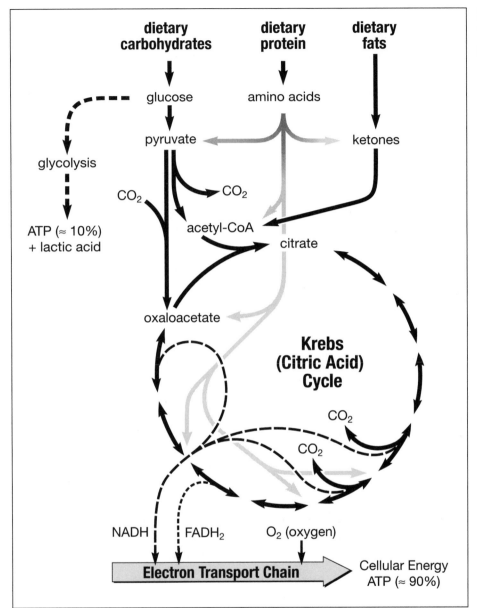

FIGURE 1-7
The Krebs
Cycle

bodies through a process known as beta-oxidation; these ketones are then further broken down into a substance called acetyl-CoA (acetyl coenzyme acetate), in which form they enter at the top of the Krebs cycle.

The primary substrates, or raw materials, for the Krebs cycle are glucose (extracted from carbohydrate foods) and the end-products of fatty acid metabolism, assisted by amino acids. Most of the glucose travels down the "left" side of the Krebs cycle (after first being transformed into pyruvate) to form a compound called oxaloacetate, while the remaining glucose combines with the fatty acids and amino acids to form acetyl CoA, which then travels down the "right" side. These substances are then further spun around the Krebs cycle with the help of additional amino acids, various enzymes, and organic acids. In a dizzying whirl of back-and-forth biochemical transmutations, acetyl CoA reacts with oxaloacetate to produce citrate (citric acid), which then reconverts back into oxaloacetate until the coenzyme intermediates are shuttled out the bottom of the Krebs cycle into the electron transport chain to complete the production of ATP energy. The intermediates so produced (the coenzymes NADH and FADH2) are passed into the electron transport chain where they undergo a further series of reactions—receiving and donating electrons down the chain—to produce energy (in the form of ATP, or adenosine triphosphate), as well as water. The presence of sufficient oxygen within the cells is essential to the success of this procedure, and, accordingly, it is known as the oxidative process (after which the Oxidative system is named).

If insufficient oxygen is being delivered to the cells—due to an overly acidic venous blood pH, or to an insufficiency of the enzyme (2–3 DPG) required to release the oxygen molecule from the red blood cell—this entire enterprise will be compromised. Alternately, an imbalance of raw materials fed to either "side" of the Krebs cycle will result in less than optimal energy production, as the two "sides" of the Krebs cycle need to balance each other out for its full energy potential to be realized. To further complicate matters, each of the two Oxidative Metabolic Types—whose energy levels are directly tied to the functioning of the Krebs cycle—require a different fuel mix. Fast Oxidizers tend to burn up glucose too rapidly; therefore they require more proteins and fats to be fed into the Krebs cycle to slow down the rate of glucose combustion. Conversely, Slow Oxidizers do not burn up glucose rapidly enough; therefore they require a higher percentage of glucose (and less protein and fats) to be fed into the Krebs cycle to fan the flames of oxidation. If either of the Oxidative types eats a diet that is inappropriately weighted in the wrong direction, the result is insufficient energy (ATP) production and metabolic imbalance. ATP is needed to carry out *all* of our biological functions. One of its primary responsibilities is protein synthesis, which itself is essential for the production of a special class of proteins known as enzymes. Enzymes are the necessary catalysts (or "spark plugs") for every single biochemical reaction in the body, from digestion to the production of neurotransmitters (brain chemicals) and hormones, and from immune function to tissue growth and DNA repair. Impaired energy production can be seen as the central malfunction that underlies *all* chronic disease. Thus we can see that feeding the body the wrong "fuel mix" for one's Metabolic Type can have far-reaching consequences, and it is precisely these negative consequences that Metabolic Typing is seeking to avoid.

Approximately 80–90% of the body's energy is generated through the Krebs cycle, in concert with the electron transport chain. The other 10–20% is produced through a less efficient process known as glycolysis, in which a portion of the glucose that would otherwise be fed into the Krebs cycle is siphoned off to create a small amount of ATP. Glycolysis can only use glucose as its raw material—very little of which can be stored in the body at any one time—whereas the Krebs cycle also uses fat, a far more abundant energy source. However, glycolysis does *not* require the presence of oxygen (defining it as an anaerobic process), unlike the Krebs cycle which can *only* function in the presence of oxygen (defining it as an aerobic process). Because the 10–20% of energy produced through glycolysis is not enough to drive our metabolic processes, it alone is insufficient to sustain human life; hence the need for oxygen for our survival. Furthermore, while the energy produced through the Krebs cycle generally burns "clean," the energy generated by glycolysis produces "smoke" in the form of lactic acid (or lactate), a potentially damaging waste product that places a serious burden on the body's detoxification systems.

All humans produce energy through the Krebs cycle, but in the Autonomic Metabolic Types this process is overshadowed by the action of the autonomic nervous system, in collaboration with the hormone (or endocrine) system. Accordingly, the Autonomic types (Sympathetics and Parasympathetics) are not so dependent on the Krebs cycle for their sense of well-being. This accounts for a phenomenon commonly noted by practitioners of Metabolic Typing. Fast Oxidizers process glucose very rapidly. After ingesting the glucose challenge drink during the Metabolic Typing protocol, the blood sugar levels of Fast Oxidizers rise then fall in a sharp curve. As their blood sugar crashes, so too does their sense of energy and well-being. Sympathetic types, however, can exhibit a similar or even identical blood sugar curve to Fast Oxidizers, but they are generally unaffected when their blood sugar levels plummet. This phenomenon, which is at first quite baffling, is simply explained by the dominance principle. Sympathetics owe their allegiance primarily to the autonomic nervous system rather than to the oxidative process, so the dynamic energy of the sympathetic branch of the nervous system carries them through a blood sugar crash that would sink a Fast Oxidizer. While we do not as yet understand the mechanics of Autonomic dominance as clearly as we do the mechanics of Oxidative dominance, the fact of its existence is quite apparent to the practitioner of Metabolic Typing. In the Autonomic types, the activity of the nervous system overrides the oxidative process; but energy production and processing—as well as providing the optimal fuel for these processes—is as central to the health of the Autonomic types as it is to the Oxidative types. It is this fundamental mechanism underlying all bodily processes that Metabolic Typing addresses, by matching each of the Metabolic Types with the correct diet designed to optimize their production of energy.

CHAPTER 2

The Practice of Metabolic Typing

HOW TO MAKE USE OF METABOLIC TYPING

Metabolic Typing was originally created as a procedure to be administered by trained healthcare professionals. This still remains the preferred method, as it allows the individual to work face-to-face with a practitioner trained and experienced in all aspects of the process, who is best able to address the specific health needs of the client. However, not everyone lives close enough to a Metabolic Typing practitioner, so a simplified *Personalized Metabolic Typing Self-Test Kit* was developed for home use. This Self-Test Kit provides enough information for the staff of Personalized Metabolic Nutrition to determine your Metabolic Type, so we can then recommend to you the appropriate diet and supplement protocol; but due to the inherent limitations of such a kit, it does not allow the practitioners to check as many metabolic markers, or assess most of the secondary imbalances, nor to go into as much detail about your specific health situation as we would be able to do in person.

For readers of this book we have created yet another option, the Self-Typing Questionnaire, which allows you to quickly determine whether you need to follow the Group I or the Group II protocols (outlined in detail in Chapter 3). This questionnaire will *not*, however, tell you your specific Metabolic Type (Fast or Slow Oxidizer; Sympathetic or Parasympathetic) for the simple reason that this level of information is beyond the scope of a questionnaire alone. However, it will suggest to you which of the two basic diet plans (Group I or Group II) is probably best suited to you. Many of you who use the Self-Typing Questionnaire may elect at a later time to go on to use the Self-Test Kit, or to find a practitioner with whom you can work in person. *The Self-Typing Questionnaire is, of necessity, not as accurate or in-depth as the other two methods,* but it will give you a place to start.

These, then, are the three ways that you, the reader, can access Metabolic Typing:

1. The Self-Typing Questionnaire
2. The Self-Test Kit
3. Consultation with a Metabolic Typing Practitioner

We will now explore these various options.

THE SELF-TYPING QUESTIONNAIRE

∾ Circle the FALSE or TRUE answer that best describes you.

∾ If neither choice fits you exactly, try to choose the one that comes closest to your tendencies.

∾ If neither choice truly applies, do not circle either.

∾ Try to answer the questions from your direct experience rather than from any preconceived ideas that you may have about the issue at hand: for example, you may believe that you should be eating low-fat foods but, in practice, fat-rich foods may actually agree with you; or you may think you are hungry between meals when, in fact, you may be eating out of habit or boredom, or because food is readily available to you—not because you are actually physically hungry.

∾ When responding to a statement phrased in the negative (e.g. "Vegetarian meals are not satisfactory to me"), a TRUE answer would mean that you agree with the statement (e.g. "Yes, it is true that vegetarian meals are not satisfactory to me"); a FALSE answer would mean that you disagree with the statement ("No, vegetarian meals are satisfactory to me").

Part One

1. My appetite at breakfast is strong   FALSE TRUE
2. My appetite at lunch is strong   FALSE TRUE

3. My appetite at dinner is strong	FALSE	TRUE
4. Going without food for four or more hours is uncomfortable	FALSE	TRUE
5. I often get hungry and need to snack between meals	FALSE	TRUE
6. I live to eat, rather than eat to live	FALSE	TRUE
7. Meat or fish at meals makes me more energetic	FALSE	TRUE
8. Vegetarian meals are not satisfactory to me	FALSE	TRUE
9. Eating meat or fatty food restores my energy	FALSE	TRUE
10. I prefer salty and/or fatty foods to sweet foods	FALSE	TRUE

Total the number of circled items above, giving *two points to each item circled* (e.g. if you circled four answers in one column, write the number 8 below in the sub-total section).

Part One Sub-Total   _____ _____

Part Two

11. Fruits alone generally do not satisfy me	FALSE	TRUE
12. Fasting is very difficult for me	FALSE	TRUE
13. Eating before bedtime improves the quality of my sleep	FALSE	TRUE
14. Orange juice in the morning does not agree with me	FALSE	TRUE
15. Coffee tends to make me feel wired or jittery	FALSE	TRUE
16. My eyes and/or nose tend to be moist	FALSE	TRUE
17. I need to urinate often during the day	FALSE	TRUE
18. I tend to cough or clear my throat fairly frequently	FALSE	TRUE
19. I prefer to sleep in, in the morning	FALSE	TRUE
20. If I cut myself, the wound heals quickly	FALSE	TRUE

Total the number of circled items above, giving *one point only to each item circled* (e.g. if you circled eight answers in one column, write the number 8 below in the sub-total section).

Part Two Sub-Total   _____ _____

Part One Sub-Total   _____ _____

GRAND TOTAL   _____ _____

∾ Add together the two sub-totals for Parts One and Two, and enter the Grand Total above.

∾ If 18 or more of your answers were FALSE, this suggests that you should follow the Group I diet (see Chapter 3 for details).

∾ If 18 or more of your answers were TRUE, this suggests that you should follow the Group II diet (see Chapter 3 for details).

∾ If you had a score of less than 18 in either column, you will probably need further testing to determine which diet group would suit you the best (see below).

Keep in mind that, due to its purely subjective nature, *a questionnaire can never be completely accurate on its own.* As you will see later on, a questionnaire is only one of several testing protocols used during an office visit with a Metabolic Typing practitioner. However, it can be used to give a general indication of a tendency toward either Group I or Group II.

THE SELF-TEST KIT

The *Personalized Metabolic Nutrition Self-Test Kit* offers the next level of involvement for individuals looking for a more in-depth analysis of their Metabolic Type. Not everyone lives in close proximity to a Metabolic Typing practitioner, or finds it convenient to go to his or her office. For these people, the *Personalized Metabolic Nutrition Self-Test Kit* has been created. The Self-Test Kit involves performing a series of simple tests in the privacy, comfort, and convenience of your own home over a period of approximately three hours. Most people find it easiest to perform the test in the morning, as it needs to done on an empty stomach, a minimum of six hours after eating any food. It does not require the presence of a healthcare professional nor, for that matter, anyone else, though some people find it helpful to have a second person assist them. Others enjoy performing the test along with a family member or friend. However, it is designed to be entirely self-contained, so that anyone can perform the test on their own. The Testing Chart that you complete during this testing period is then faxed or mailed to the Personalized

Metabolic Nutrition office, where it will be analyzed. A report will then be faxed or mailed back to you informing you of your Metabolic Type, and outlining the diet and supplement recommendations that are specific to your Metabolic Type.

The *Personalized Metabolic Self-Test Kit* contains the following items:

- A glucometer (blood glucose meter) and test strips
- A lancet holder and lancets
- Glucose and protein challenge powders
- Alcohol swabs and pH papers
- Step-by-step written instructions
- A Questionnaire, Medical History Form, and a Waiver
- A Personalized Metabolic Self-Test Chart

(Please refer to Resources for information on how to order the *Personalized Metabolic Nutrition Self-Test Kit.*)

Consulting with a Metabolic Typing Practitioner

At the time of this writing there is a growing but still limited number of healthcare practitioners (including medical doctors, osteopaths, naturopaths, chiropractors, nutritionists, acupuncturists, dentists, etc.) trained in Metabolic Typing. There are numerous advantages to working with such individuals. They are able to perform more in-depth testing than the Self-Typing Questionnaire or the Self-Test Kit permit; they can spend more time discussing your particular health needs and concerns; they can more precisely target their nutritional recommendations to your specific health conditions; and they can establish an ongoing relationship with you to allow them to monitor your progress over time. (Please refer to "Understanding the Testing Protocols of Metabolic Typing" in Appendix A for an in-depth exploration of the testing methodologies used in our own nutrition clinic and by other Metabolic Typing practitioners during individual consultations. Refer to Resources for information on how to locate a practitioner of Metabolic Typing in your area).

METABOLIC TYPES:
DISTINGUISHING CHARACTERISTICS

The following list of distinguishing characteristics is not intended to be definitive, and it describes general characteristics only. *Exceptions are commonly found in all of these categories,* including in the disease conditions shown. Some of these characteristics apply more to either the Autonomic or Oxidative types. As with all of the typing parameters, these characteristics need to be seen within the context of the other testing methods. Very few people are pure types (i.e. 100% one particular Metabolic Type); most are a mixture of types, to one degree or another, but with one type predominating. Various lifestyle factors can also affect some of these characteristics: for example, a Group II individual who, by tendency, has good digestion and sleeps well may suffer from indigestion or insomnia due to stress.

Group I *Slow Oxidizers* *Sympathetics*	Group II *Fast Oxidizers* *Parasympathetics*
Tall & lean	Short & stocky
Pale ears	Red ears
Large pupils	Small-to-medium pupils
Dry eyes & mouth	Moist eyes & mouth
Dry throat	Phlegm in throat
Slow healer	Fast healer
Sleeps poorly	Sleeps well
Wakes up easily	Likes to sleep in
Poor digestion	Good digestion
Infrequently hungry	Frequently hungry
Infrequent urination	Frequent urination
Constipation	Diarrhea
Syndrome X	Diabetes (Type II)
High blood pressure	Low blood pressure
High body temperature	Low body temperature

Slow respiratory rate	Fast respiratory rate
Long breath-hold (over 50 seconds)	Short breath-hold (under 50 seconds)
Migraines	Asthma
Hyperthyroid	Hypothyroid
Goal oriented*	Procrastinates/*laissez faire**
Solitary*	Social*
Hyper*	Calm*

Asterisks indicate predominantly Autonomic system characteristics (applying to Sympathetics and Parasympathetics, respectively) that do not necessarily apply to the Oxidative types (Fast and Slow Oxidizers).

CHAPTER 3

Diets for the Metabolic Types

SO WHAT *DO* I EAT?

As we have seen, the linchpin of the Metabolic Typing model is the theory of the two dominance systems, the Oxidative and the Autonomic. One *or* the other of these dominance systems will be more active than the other system in any given individual; and within that particular dominance system, one of the two sub-types will best characterize each individual. The Oxidative types are Fast or Slow Oxidizers; the Autonomic types are Sympathetics or Parasympathetics.

We have also seen how, within each dominance system, there is both an acid and an alkaline blood type. In the Oxidative System, the Fast Oxidizer is the acid blood type, and the Slow Oxidizer is the alkaline blood type. In the Autonomic System, the Sympathetic is the acid blood type and the Parasympathetic is the alkaline blood type. The two acid blood types—the Fast Oxidizer and the Sympathetic—share the quality of rapidly oxidizing (or burning up) carbohydrates, while the two alkaline blood types—the Slow Oxidizer and the Parasympathetic—share the quality of more slowly oxidizing carbohydrates.

Acid	Alkaline
Fast Oxidizer	Slow Oxidizer
Sympathetic	Parasympathetic

When it comes to dietary recommendations, however, our four Metabolic Types are divided up into two different groups, Groups I and II. It would seem logical that we would put the two acid types in one diet group and the two alkaline types in another. However, what we actually end up with is the acid member of one dominance system sharing the same diet as the alkaline member of the opposite dominance system.

When it comes to diet, the Metabolic Types are, therefore, divided up as follows:

Group I	Group II
Slow Oxidizer (alkaline)	Fast Oxidizer (acid)
Sympathetic (acid)	Parasympathetic (alkaline)

Why would two Metabolic Types with opposite pHs share the same diet? The reason for this lies in the phenomenon we have mentioned several times previously: with a few exceptions, *the same foods affect members of the two dominance systems in opposite ways.* In other words, foods that acidify the Oxidative types (Fast and Slow Oxidizers), alkalize the Autonomic types (Sympathetics and Parasympathetics); and foods that alkalize the Oxidative types, acidify the Autonomic types. Why exactly it works this way is unknown at the present time, but clearly the key lies in how the different dominance systems function. Whatever the mechanics behind it, however, this phenomenon has been well documented over the years by those working within the field of Metabolic Typing. This key observation sets the Metabolic Typing practitioner aside from any other nutritionist working with the pH of foods.

The conventional approach takes a static or absolutist view: that the pH effect of a given food is dependent on the inherent qualities of the food itself—though this pH effect is not necessarily the same as the pH of the food itself (for example, citrus fruits are inherently acidic, but in the conventional view are generally believed to be alkaline forming in the body). By contrast, Metabolic Typing takes a fluid or relativistic view: that the pH effect of a given food is a result of the *interaction* between the inherent qualities of the food itself *and* the metabolism of the person eating it. It *is* true that if you take a food substance into a laboratory, reduce it to ash, and analyze the ash, the ash will have a characteristic pH. However, that inherent pH does not itself determine how that same food will affect any given individual. It

Blood Versus Urine and Saliva pHs

Conventional nutritional wisdom holds that any particular food will have the *same* pH effect in anyone who eats it. Thus it is commonly said that protein foods (especially animal proteins) are generally acid forming, and that fruits and vegetables are generally alkaline forming. But, in the world of Metabolic Typing—where *blood* is being used as the primary pH marker—this would *only* be true of the two Autonomic types. For the two Oxidative types, the opposite would apply: most animal proteins would be alkaline forming, and most fruits and vegetables would be acid forming. Almost all other nutritionists who work with pHs use urine and/or saliva—not blood—as their primary marker. This is simply for ease of access. Urine and saliva pHs can easily be gathered and measured, whereas blood pH cannot. However, not only are urine and saliva much more changeable and, therefore, less reliable as metabolic markers than blood pH, but *urine generally runs opposite to blood pH.* Saliva, by contrast, generally parallels the blood. The fact that this is only *generally* so, and not always so, is due to multiple and complex metabolic factors, as well as the changeability of urine and saliva pHs. It is much more critical to the body's metabolic functioning that the blood be kept within a more narrow pH range than the urine and saliva. So, given that urine generally runs opposite to the blood pH, our example above would have to be inverted if urine—and not blood—were the primary marker used to infer the pH reaction to foods. If animal foods are acid forming to the urine, they would typically (though not always) be alkaline forming to the blood, which is the response found among the Oxidative, not Autonomic types.

will alkalize members of one dominance system, but acidify members of the opposite system.

Although this idea can be a bit tricky to grasp conceptually, it actually goes along with common sense. It is a perfect example of "different strokes for different folks," and it also reflects the old adage that "one man's meat is another man's poison." Furthermore, it reinforces the concept of biochemical individuality that we have referred to previously: even though our component parts are all the same, *we are not all the same in terms of our biochemical responses,* just as we do not all respond emotionally in the same way to the same situation.

So what are the two food groups, and how do we determine which foods are right for which Metabolic Types? Essentially, we base this on how foods

affect the pH of the blood. The research into this process was originally conducted by George Watson, Ph.D.—the formulator of the Oxidative System—
and was later corroborated by his follower Rudolf Wiley.[1] Wiley took fasting
blood pH readings, then fed his research subjects three-ounce portions of
particular foods. A second blood pH reading was then taken to see how the
food affected the blood pH. Based on this research, lists were drawn up detailing which foods moved the blood in the acid or alkaline direction.

We have seen that foods affect members of the two dominance systems in
opposite ways. So, foods that acidify the Oxidative types (Fast and Slow Oxidizers) alkalize the Autonomic types (Sympathetics and Parasympathetics).
Let us use the humble tomato as an example. The tomato was found to be
acidifying to the Oxidative types. For the Slow Oxidizer, who is overly alkaline, this would be desirable as it would help to counteract his or her alkaline
tendency by acidifying the blood. But for the Fast Oxidizer, who is already too
acid, the tomato would tend to exacerbate his or her condition. Therefore, the
tomato would be desirable for the Slow Oxidizer but undesirable for the Fast
Oxidizer—at least as a staple food.

For our two Autonomic types, however, the tomato would have the opposite effect: it would be alkalizing. This would be desirable for the Sympathetic,
who runs on the acid side, but undesirable for the Parasympathetic, who
already runs on the alkaline side. Therefore, the tomato is seen as a Group I
food, because it is desirable for our two Group I types: the Slow Oxidizer and
the Sympathetic. Conversely, it would be contraindicated as a staple food for
our two Group II types: the Fast Oxidizer and the Parasympathetic.

Let us take another example: spinach. Spinach was found to be alkaline
forming to the Oxidative types. For the Slow Oxidizer, who is overly alkaline, this would be undesirable as it would further exacerbate his or her alkaline tendencies. But for the Fast Oxidizer, who is too acid, spinach would
tend to counteract his or her acid tendency by helping to alkalize the blood.
Therefore, spinach would be undesirable for the Slow Oxidizer but desirable
for the Fast Oxidizer. For our two Autonomic types, spinach would have the
opposite effect: it would be acidifying. This would be undesirable for the
Sympathetic, who already runs on the acid side, but desirable for the Parasympathetic, who runs on the alkaline side. Therefore, spinach is seen as a Group
II food, because it is desirable for our two Group II types: the Fast Oxidizer

and the Parasympathetic. Conversely, it would be contraindicated—at least on a regular basis—for our two Group I types: the Slow Oxidizer and the Sympathetic. Let's hope Popeye was a Group II type!

Now, both these foods—tomatoes and spinach—are normally considered to be universally healthy foods. However, as we have seen, they are much healthier for some Metabolic Types than for others. The further out of balance an individual is, or the more extreme an example of their particular Metabolic Type they are, the more important it is that they stick closely to the foods that are best suited to their group. Thus we can see the importance of knowing your Metabolic Type when selecting your food.

Based on Watson and Wiley's research, and the subsequent clinical experience of myself and Bill Wolcott, we are able to summarize the two food groups as follows:

Group I
Slow Oxidizers (alkaline)
Sympathetics (acid)

Lower in protein and fats
Higher in complex carbohydrates

Group I foods will *acidify* the Slow Oxidizers (who are too alkaline) and *alkalize* the Sympathetics (who are too acid); both will thereby be brought closer to the ideal venous blood pH of 7.46.

Group II
Fast Oxidizers (acid)
Parasympathetics (alkaline)

Higher in protein and fats
Lower in complex carbohydrates

Group II foods will *alkalize* the Fast Oxidizers (who are too acid) and *acidify* the Parasympathetics (who are too alkaline); both will thereby be brought closer to the ideal venous blood pH of 7.46.

FIGURE 3-1

How Foods Affect the Oxidative and Autonomic Systems

There is both an acid and alkaline blood type within each dominance system:

Acid Blood	Alkaline Blood
Fast Oxidizers *and* *Sympathetics*	*Slow Oxidizers* *and* *Parasympathetics*

When it comes to diet, however, the dominance systems react oppositely:

Group I Foods	Group II Foods
are *higher in complex carbs* *and* *lower in proteins and fats.*	*are* *higher in proteins and fats* *and* *lower in complex carbs.*

acidify the Oxidizers	*alkalize the Oxidizers*
alkalize the Autonomics	*acidify the Autonomics*

Group I foods will *acidify* the overly alkaline Slow Oxidizers, and *alkalize* the overly acid Sympathetics	Group II foods will *alkalize* the overly acid Fast Oxidizers, and *acidify* the overly alkaline Parasympathetics
Both will thereby be brought closer to the ideal venous blood pH of 7.46	Both will thereby be brought closer to the ideal venous blood pH of 7.46

Group I Foods

It will be noted that the Group I types require less protein and fats than the Group II types. They also do best on the less rich proteins, which are generally proteins with a lower fat content, and which are typically lighter in color. Therefore, Group I proteins (see Figure 3-2) should be primarily in the form of the lighter meats (white-meat chicken and turkey, lean cuts of pork) and the less oily fish (primarily white fish).

The sluggish metabolism of the Slow Oxidizer is further slowed down by too much protein and fat. However, complex carbohydrates provide the quick-burning fuel needed to speed up their oxidation rate, or stoke their energy furnaces. By contrast, Sympathetics are running on the nervous energy of the more dynamic, or *hyper,* branch of the autonomic nervous system.

Too much protein and fat only serve as gasoline on the fire of their already over-revved metabolism, but complex carbohydrates put on the brakes so that their energy production is slowed down and made more even. Thus we can see that complex carbohydrates have opposite effects on our two Group I types: they speed up the sluggish Slow Oxidizer, but slow down the speedy Sympathetic. This points back to the key principle of our two dominance systems: foods affect the Oxidative and the Autonomic types in precisely different ways.

It should be emphasized that Group I types thrive on complex carbohydrates, *not* simple carbohydrates. Complex carbohydrates include whole grains and whole grain products, as well as fruits and vegetables. But we live in a culture that is infatuated with *simple* carbohydrates. Simple carbohydrates include sugar and *all* sweeteners (with the exception of the herbal sweetener stevia), as well as white rice and all foods made from refined (white) flour. The list of white flour products is very long indeed, and includes white bread, pasta, pizza, bagels, pretzels, muffins, cakes, pies, and cookies—in other words most of our "comfort foods"! Fortunately, many health food stores now sell whole grain versions of all of these foods and, although they are usually still somewhat processed, they represent a quantum leap beyond mainstream supermarket fare. It is true that their prices may be somewhat higher, but your health is worth a few extra pennies on the dollar.

All grains are fine for the Group I types, but whole wheat is generally the best grain of all. This often surprises people who have been involved with natural foods for some time, as many health authorities vilify wheat, due to its high allergy-promoting quotient. However, for the Group I types, wheat is very balancing: it acidifies the overly alkaline Slow Oxidizers, and alkalizes the overly acidic Sympathetics. Only in cases where there is an outright wheat allergy or gluten intolerance should wheat be avoided by the Group I types. All fruits are also acceptable, as are most vegetables, with an emphasis on leafy greens and cruciferous vegetables (the cabbage family, which includes broccoli and Brussels sprouts). All of the nightshades (potatoes, tomatoes, eggplants, peppers) are also Group I foods. However, whole grains, starchy vegetables, and sweet fruits should be limited in situations where weight loss or blood sugar problems are a concern, or in individuals with cancer (as these foods rapidly convert into glucose, and excess glucose fuels the expansion of fat cells and tumors).

Figure 3-2   Group I Foods *for Slow Oxidizers & Sympathetics*

PROTEINS			
Meat	**Seafood**	**Dairy**	**Misc. Proteins**
Eat light meats & *avoid dark meats:*	*Eat white fish &* *shellfish only:*	*Limited use of low-* *or non-fat dairy only:*	eggs
pork (lean)	catfish	cheese	*In moderation:*
poultry breast	cod	cottage cheese	beans (dried)
	flounder	milk	tempeh
Minimize:	haddock	yogurt	tofu
organ meats	halibut		
red meats	perch		
	scrod		
	sole		
	trout		
	tuna (white)		
	In moderation:		
	crab		
	crayfish		
	lobster		
	shrimp		
	other shellfish		
	Minimize:		
	oily fish		

- ~ Eat protein every day at two or more meals, with plenty of fresh vegetables.
- ~ Eat three regular meals per day; rotate your food selections to avoid eating the same foods every day.
- ~ Eat organic meats and produce whenever possible; avoid all processed foods.
- ~ Use unrefined, non-hydrogenated oils only, preferably organically grown and cold-pressed.
- ~ Bake, broil, grill, or poach animal foods; do not overcook or blacken.
- ~ Emphasize a variety of leafy greens, both lightly cooked and in salads.

Nuts and seeds should only be eaten in moderation, with almonds being the nut of choice for the Group I types. Oils should also be used sparingly, with olive oil (preferably organic, cold-pressed, extra virgin olive oil) being the best all-round culinary and salad oil. Coconut oil can be used sparingly for cooking and baking, but only in its unrefined form. Eggs are an excellent protein source, but care should be taken to purchase organically produced eggs, preferably from free range chickens. Dairy products should generally be of the lower fat variety. There are certain vegetables that should be min-

CARBS				FATS
Grains	**Veggies**		**Fruit**	**Oils/Nuts**
All are OK, but whole wheat is best:	*Emphasize the following:*		*All are OK including, but not limited to:*	*Use sparingly:*
amaranth	beets	lettuce	apples	almonds
barley	broccoli	onions	apricots	almond butter
buckwheat	Brussels spouts	parsley	bananas (ripe)	tahini
corn	cabbage	peppers	berries	flax oil
kamut	chard	potatoes	cherries	olive oil
millet	corn	radishes	citrus	
quinoa	cucumber	sprouts (any)	grapes	*In moderation:*
rice (brown)	eggplant	squash (soft)	melons	coconut oil
rye	garlic	tomatoes	peaches	sesame oil
spelt	jicama	turnip	pears	all other nuts
wheat	kale	yam	pineapple	pumpkin seeds
	leafy greens	zucchini	plums	sesame seeds
Minimize:				sunflower seeds
oats	*Minimize:*			
	artichoke	lentils		*Minimize:*
	asparagus	mushrooms		butter
	avocado	olives		fatty foods
	carrots	peas		salty foods
	cauliflower	spinach		
	celery	winter squash		

- ∾ Breads and other flour products should be made from whole grains.
- ∾ Drink 2 glasses of filtered or distilled water on arising; drink a total of 6-8 glasses per day.
- ∾ Minimize alcohol (especially hard liquor) and coffee; completely avoid sodas (diet or regular).
- ∾ Avoid all sugar and artificial sweeteners (*NutraSweet*, etc.); use stevia, xylitol, or raw honey.
- ∾ Restrict salt intake; use unrefined (gray/beige) sea salts, such as Celtic, Eden, Mediterranean, or Real Salt.

imized or avoided, such as avocado, artichoke, asparagus and spinach (see Figure 3-2). Salty and fatty foods should be restricted, and red meat should be eaten only occasionally (preferably no more than once or twice a week).

The Group I diet is substantially lower in fat than the Group II diet, and it has much in common with the low-fat diet recommendations made by mainstream health authorities. However, a word of caution is needed concerning foods marketed as low-fat. The taste and feel of fat is very compelling to most of us—and with good reason, as some fat is vital to our health and well-being—so the marketers of low-fat foods have to find a substitute that will satisfy the taste buds. The easiest substitute is sugar and other refined carbs; therefore most so-called low-fat foods are a sham. Yes, they have a lower fat content, but they are composed of empty calories (i.e. devoid of substantive nutritional content) that are themselves quite fattening! This includes frozen yogurt, which converts an intrinsically healthy food into a sugar bomb; and sugar itself, which comes disguised in many forms so as to elude the notice of all but the most observant consumers, usually in words ending in *-ose* (sucrose, fructose, maltose, etc.) or *-ol* (such as sorbitol).

The Group I diet is easily adaptable for vegetarians. Vegetarian diets are almost always low in protein and high in carbohydrates because plant foods are predominantly composed of carbohydrates, even the higher protein plant foods like grains and legumes. The grains with the highest protein content (wheat, amaranth, quinoa) only contain about 15% protein; most of the remaining 85% is carbohydrates. There are a few plant "superfoods" that have a much higher protein content—such as algae (spirulina, chlorella, blue-green algae, etc.), nutritional yeast, and bee pollen—but it would be impractical to eat them in anything other than relatively small quantities (and strict vegans may also argue whether algae and pollen should truly be considered plant or animal foods). Group I vegetarians would, however, need to eat a higher proportion of legumes than is generally recommended for Group I types in order to acquire sufficient protein.

Frequently, Group I types do not feel especially hungry in the morning, and often do not bother with much breakfast, preferring instead a cup or two of coffee and, perhaps, a piece of toast, a muffin, or a piece of fruit. However, breakfast is a very important meal to jumpstart the metabolism in the morning after a night of fasting (hence the origin of the word "break-fast"). So, even if the meal is light, such as a protein and fruit smoothie, something with more nutritional substance than coffee and white toast should be eaten. Because Group I types tend not to especially notice their hunger—Slow Oxidizers, because they take a long time to burn up their carbohydrates; Sympathetics, because they are running on nervous system energy—they tend to forget or skip meals. But, even though they are much more able to do so than the Group II types, it is nonetheless important that they eat three regular meals to replenish their energy reserves, to keep their blood sugar stable, and to ensure that they consume enough volume of food to receive a sufficient quantity of required daily nutrients. The suggested protein foods should be eaten at least twice a day, as protein is still important to the Group I types; it is simply that they need less of it, and in less rich forms, than the Group II types.

Group II Foods

Group II types require a much higher amount of protein and fat than their Group I counterparts. This makes their diet somewhat "politically incorrect" in today's low-fat climate. Often our Group II clients are either shocked or relieved (or both!) when we show them the list of foods we want them to eat (see Figure 3-3). Many fear their cholesterol levels will soar and that they will put on weight, but the opposite is frequently the case. When a person is eating the right foods for their Metabolic Type, their blood lipids (cholesterol and triglycerides) and weight tend to normalize. Usually, the noticeable increase in their energy level is enough to convince them that they are indeed on the right diet!

Fast Oxidizers combust, or burn up, carbohydrates rapidly. If the energy so produced is not used up in the short term through some kind of physical activity, it will tend to turn either into excess serum cholesterol and triglycerides or body fat (adipose tissue). Protein and good quality fats slow down this process, and so they allow energy to be generated in a slower and more even fashion. By contrast, Parasympathetics tend to have somewhat sluggish systems, and this is exacerbated in the Autonomic types by a diet too high in carbohydrates (this is exactly the opposite effect that we have noted in the Oxidative types). Protein and good quality fats will, conversely, tend to stimulate the more energetic sympathetic branch of the nervous system in the Parasympathetics, thereby moving them toward a balance point, speeding up their metabolism and improving their energy levels.

The Group II diet emphasizes protein foods and good quality fats, which should be the central focus of each meal. Because fats typically come "built in" to protein foods, simply eating enough protein foods generally ensures that you will also be getting adequate amounts of fats. Optimally, this would also extend to the between-meal snacks that the Group II types often require to keep their energy levels up. Any and all protein foods are suitable for the Group II types, but they do best with darker meats (red meat, dark-meat

FIGURE 3-3   Group II Foods *for Fast Oxidizers & Parasympathetics*

PROTEINS			
Meat	**Seafood**	**Dairy**	**Misc. Proteins**
All are OK but emphasize dark meats:	*All are OK but emphasize oily fish:*	*All whole milk is OK (cow, goat, sheep):*	eggs
			beans (dried)
			lentils
beef	anchovies	cheese	tempeh
lamb	fish eggs/roe	cottage cheese	tofu
liver	herring	cream	
organ meats	mackerel	milk	
poultry (dark)	salmon	yogurt	
red meat (any)	sardines		
steak	tuna (dark)		
	abalone		
	crab		
	lobster		
	oyster		
	scallop		
	shrimp		
	other shellfish		

- ❧ Eat three regular meals per day, with a couple of snacks as needed; do not eat the same foods every day.
- ❧ Eat protein with every meal; never eat carbohydrates alone.
- ❧ Eat organic meats and produce whenever possible; avoid all processed foods.
- ❧ Use unrefined, non-hydrogenated oils only, preferably organically grown and cold-pressed.
- ❧ Bake, broil, grill, or poach animal foods; do not overcook or blacken.

chicken and poultry) and the oilier fish (salmon, sardines, herring, dark tuna, etc.) and with proteins that are higher in a particular substance called purines. Purines are nitrogen-based compounds that orchestrate protein synthesis and are especially important for energy production in the Group II types. They are most concentrated in organ meats, sardines, anchovies, and fish eggs (caviar or roe), and are moderately high in shellfish and red meat, as well as lentils, spinach, and many of the other Group II vegetables. Generally, as a society, we do not tend to be attracted to organ meats (liver, kid-

CARBS			FATS
Grains	**Veggies**	**Fruit**	**Oils/Nuts**
All are OK, except wheat, including:	*Emphasize the following:*	*Only have the following:* apples (tart)	*All oils, nuts & seeds are OK, including::*

amaranth
barley
buckwheat
corn
kamut
millet
oats
quinoa
rice (brown)
rye
spelt
	artichoke green beans
	asparagus mushrooms
	avocado olives
	carrots peas
	cauliflower spinach
	celery winter squash
	
	In moderation:
	chard
	kale salad greens
		(Granny Smith,
		  Pippin)
		banana (firm)
		pears (firm)
		  (Bosc, D'Anjou)
		
		In moderation:
		apricots
		blueberries
		other berries
		plums
			butter
			nut butters
			tahini
			oils (coconut
			  flax
			  olive
			  sesame)
			nuts/seeds
			  (almonds
			  brazils
			  cashews

Avoid:
wheat and all
by-products
	Minimize:
	beets
	broccoli potatoes
	Brussels sprouts soft squashes
	cabbage sprouts
	eggplant tomatoes
	garlic turnip
	mustard greens zucchini
	onions
		Minimize:
		citrus fruits
		grapes
		sweet fruits
		
		Avoid:
		all fruit juices
		vinegar
			filbert
			  macadamia
			  peanuts
			  pecans
			  pumpkin
			  sesame
			  sunflower
			  walnuts)

- ❧ Breads and flour products should be made from rye, brown rice, spelt, or other non-wheat whole grains.
- ❧ Drink 2 glasses of filtered or distilled water on arising; drink a total of 6-8 glasses per day.
- ❧ Minimize alcohol (especially hard liquor) and coffee; avoid fruit juices and all sodas (diet or regular).
- ❧ Avoid all sugar and artificial sweeteners (*NutraSweet*, etc.); use stevia or xylitol instead.
- ❧ Use unrefined (gray/beige) sea salt, such as Celtic, Eden, Mediterranean, or Real Salt.

neys, etc.), and they are something of an acquired taste; but for a Group II type they are some of the best of all possible foods. However, they should come preferably from organically raised, free-range animals, to avoid the concentration of toxins that can otherwise occur in organ meats from factory-farmed animals. Optimally, some purine foods should be part of the Group II daily diet.

Eggs, though not high in purines, are also an excellent source of high quality protein, and can be eaten liberally. Try to find organic eggs from free-range chickens to avoid the contaminants from antibiotics and pesticides commonly found in commercially produced eggs. Whole (full-fat) dairy products should be chosen over the low-fat variety, and butter can be used in moderation. Wherever possible, use raw, organically produced dairy products; those from free-range (pasture fed) dairy cattle are infinitely superior to their commercial versions, not just in terms of the absence of contaminants, but also in considerably superior nutrient density and fatty acid profile. However, if weight is an issue, it may be necessary to limit the intake of dairy products.

Whole grains can be used as adjunct foods—that is, as side dishes, not as the featured dish. However, the one big exception is wheat, which is strongly contraindicated for the Group II types. Wheat and wheat products—including whole wheat—are very acid forming for the already overly acid Fast Oxidizers, and very alkaline forming for the already overly alkaline Parasympathetics; in other words, they push these Metabolic Types in precisely the wrong directions. Unfortunately for the Group II types, wheat products are ubiquitous in our culture, and it takes some attentiveness to avoid them, particularly when eating out in restaurants. Part of the problem with wheat for the Group II types is that it has been so heavily hybridized over the centuries; its older cousins, spelt and kamut, do not create the same problems for the Group II types. Breads made from whole rye, brown rice, millet, or other whole grains; rye, oat, or brown rice crackers; and pastas made from brown rice, corn, or quinoa can be used in moderation; but even these should be a relatively small part of the diet, as they are high carbohydrate foods. In fact, once a grain has been ground into flour, even a whole grain flour, it converts into glucose much more rapidly in the body than would the whole grain itself.

While the range of protein foods is unlimited on the Group II diet, the vegetable and fruit selection is somewhat limited. All the nightshades (potatoes, tomatoes, eggplants, peppers) and cruciferous vegetables (the cabbage family, including broccoli) should be minimized or avoided—the one exception being cauliflower. The vegetables to emphasize include spinach, carrots, celery, asparagus, artichoke, avocado, cauliflower, and winter squashes, with moderate use of other leafy greens, such as chard, kale, and salad greens.

The Group II fruits are the less sweet fruits, typically more readily available in the fall and winter months. These include the more tart apples (Granny Smiths, Pippins), firmer pears (Bosc, D'Anjou), and less ripe bananas (with green tips). Berries (especially blueberries, and to a lesser extent strawberries and raspberries) and some of the other less sweet fruits can be used in moderation, when they are in season. However, fruit should never play a large part in the Group II diet, and should not be eaten more than once, or perhaps twice, a day. Nuts and seeds are excellent snack foods for the Group II types, and any good quality, unrefined oils can be used. Olive oil (preferably organic, cold-pressed, extra virgin) is the best all-round oil for salads and light sautéing, but coconut oil (organic and unrefined) is the best oil for cooking and baking due to its high smoke point, its stability when subjected to heat. Coconut oil (sometimes also known as coconut butter) is highly nutritious, and although it is made up almost entirely of saturated fat, it is primarily in the form of short- and medium-chain triglycerides that the body uses for energy, rather than stores as body fat.

The Group II types, especially the Fast Oxidizers, tend to easily get hungry between meals, especially when not consuming enough purine-dense foods. It is very important that Group II types eat regular meals, and they should *always* eat something when hungry. Fast Oxidizers are especially prone to blood sugar crashes if they do not get food on a timely basis, and this phenomenon can be very detrimental to their health over time—possibly setting the stage for hypoglycemia (low blood sugar) or even adult-onset diabetes. Group II types should feel free to eat snacks between meals, but preferably protein- and/or fat-rich snacks, such as cottage cheese, half an apple with a hunk of cheese, a piece of celery spread with nut butter, tuna or sardines, half an avocado, or a handful of seeds and nuts. Avoid eating carbohydrate foods on their own (such as crackers, popcorn, or chips), as these will not provide sustained energy.

It should be noted that it is difficult to be a vegetarian on the Group II diet. As already mentioned, vegetarian diets are inherently higher in carbohydrates than in protein, and very low in purine-containing foods. If a vegetarian is willing to modify his or her diet to include eggs, dairy products, and fish, then it is possible to eat a semi-vegetarian diet that speaks to their metabolic needs. But strict Group II vegetarians are faced with a difficult choice, between sticking to their principles and compromising their health. Younger Group II types might appear to do well on vegetarian diets, but problems with energy and digestion, and possibly more serious ailments, are likely to show up in the middle and later years.

Oils

We will be looking at oils and fats in more detail in Chapter 6. For now, though, we must stress how important it is to use good quality oils. Most oils sold in supermarkets are extracted with toxic solvents, then filtered, refined, purified, and bleached. This produces oils of a very poor quality that do not contribute to our good health. They are also generally packaged in clear glass or plastic bottles, which let in light, and are kept at room temperature, which lets in heat. Light and heat, along with oxygen, are the great enemies of oil, and hasten its spoilage or rancidity, producing toxic substances in the oil. Other oils—used in almost all commercial baked goods, fast foods (such as French fries), and margarine—are partially hydrogenated, a process that produces *trans* fatty acids (*trans* is short for transformed), dangerously toxic substances that have been implicated in many degenerative diseases, ranging from arthritis to lung cancer to heart disease.[2] At the very least, these oils place an undue burden on your liver, contribute to the inflammatory process, and seriously interfere with proper cellular functioning, including the functioning of brain cells. *They are, arguably, the very worst food substances you can put in your body,* so you should try to avoid completely *any* food that contains partially hydrogenated oils or *trans* fats.

Furthermore, oils from crops that are not organically grown tend to concentrate the pesticides and herbicides used on the crop. Therefore, whenever possible, use organically grown oils that have been cold-pressed (not subjected to damaging heat), and are not refined or purified. Olive oil should be extra virgin (i.e. from the first pressing). In general, the omega-6 oils (corn, safflower, sunflower, and soy) should be minimized or avoided, as they tend to contribute to an imbalance in the ratio between omega-6 and omega-3 fatty acids, which optimally should be in the 4:1 to 2:1 range.[3] Liberal use of the omega-6 oils, which are the most commonly used salad and culinary oils, upsets this ratio, which can contribute to numerous inflammatory conditions—ranging from arthritis to cardiovascular disease—and may even be implicated in the development of some forms of cancer. Moderate or occasional use of the more benign omega-6 oils—such as sesame or grapeseed oil—is fine, but, in general, enough omega-6 fatty acids are derived from foods such as nuts, seeds, whole grains, leafy green vegetables, and animal foods. Canola oil (from rapeseed) has become quite popular in recent years, and is heavily marketed as an omega-3 oil. In fact, its omega-3 content is quite modest (10% or less), and often does not survive the refining process that this oil is almost inevitably subjected to.[4] More disturbing is the fact that most of the canola oil sold in the US is from genetically engineered crops. Because of these factors, we do not recommend regular use of canola oil.

Buy Organic

Commercially grown foods are subjected to a wide array of chemical fertilizers, pesticides, herbicides, and fungicides. Some of these chemicals inevitably end up in the food itself. Agribusiness interests claim that most crops contain only very small traces of these substances, and that they are safe. It is true that the levels of these chemicals ingested from any given food is usually small, but safe they are definitely not! The body has difficulty eliminating many of these compounds, and they tend to accumulate in the tissues; thus, small amounts ingested over several decades cease to be small amounts, and the interactions between the hundreds of different chemicals used have never been tested. It is well known that mixing different household cleaning agents together can be extremely dangerous, so it is not far-fetched to assume similar problems may exist with agricultural chemicals. Several of them have already been directly linked to cancer, which is at almost epidemic levels in our society. The long-term effect of combining the several hundred agricultural chemicals currently in use is completely unknown.

Children are especially susceptible to the toxic effects of these chemicals. The Environmental Working Group in Washington DC has estimated that millions of children in the U.S. receive up to 35% of their entire lifetime exposure to potentially carcinogenic pesticides by the time they are five years old, a time at which the developing nervous system is especially vulnerable. Chemical residues on agricultural products have risen astronomically in the last fifty years, over 100,000% from 1945 to 1990! Is it a coincidence that the rate of childhood cancers, especially leukemia and brain cancer, has risen over 20% from 1975 to 1996?[5] We are playing Russian roulette with our health and the health of our children if we subsist on a diet of chemicalized foods, however small the amount may be in any particular isolated food. Organically grown food, which is what the human race has consumed for its entire history until the last century, should be seen as a necessity and a basic right, not a luxury for the privileged.

Furthermore, these same agricultural chemicals are a major contributor to groundwater contamination and airborne pollution. Our chemical farming practices have wreaked havoc on the ecology of the planet. We all give lip-service to ecological concerns, but buying organic is a way to make a real difference in this crucial arena, as we are "voting with our dollars." In addition to producing higher quality food, organic farming actually improves the quality of the soil over time, whereas chemical farming savagely depletes it, leaving a legacy of ever more barren soil for generations to come.

Organically grown food is available in most natural food stores, and is more and more making its way into mainstream supermarkets. It will do so to the degree that there is a perceived demand. So make sure that you voice that demand to the manager of your local supermarket. If you have a farmers' market in your area, please patronize it. You get the benefit of the freshest produce possible, often at prices lower than those in the stores, and have the distinct pleasure of helping to support your local family farmers, an endangered species who are almost as much in need of our support as endangered wild animals.

It is equally important to buy meats from organically reared, free-range animals. Again, the quality of the meat is superior, especially in pasture fed (grass fed) animals; it is free of the hormones and antibiotics widely used in conventional animal husbandry, and free of the pesticides ingested through the animal feed—all of which tend to accumulate in the fatty tissue of the animal. The fatty acid profile is also much more beneficial in the milk or meat of pasture fed cattle, including much higher amounts of CLA (conjugated linoleic acid), a recently discovered fatty acid that is only minimally present (if at all) in feed-lot cows, which are fed an unnatural diet of corn and soy. CLA has received a lot of attention for its wide range of health benefits, which include the ability to facilitate the conversion of body fat into lean muscle tissue, enhance immune function, balance the blood sugar, and protect against cancer and heart disease.[6] Furthermore, by purchasing free-range animal products, you will be supporting humane farming practices, rather than the cruelty that is all too common in factory farming.

Milk and Dairy Products

Wherever possible, milk (and all other dairy products) should be used in their traditional raw form, preferably from free range, grass-fed cows that have not been dosed with bovine growth hormones or antibiotics. Raw milk is nutritionally superior to commercial milk, as pasteurization destroys valuable enzymes, beneficial bacteria, and many other nutrients in milk, while homogenization (the breaking of milk fat into tiny particles) releases a substance (xanthine oxidase) that has been implicated in damaging the walls of the arteries.[7] These processing methods make it difficult for the body to properly digest dairy products, and almost certainly contribute to the widespread phenomenon of dairy allergies, which are almost unknown in cultures where raw milk products are consumed. Note that dairy products labeled "organic" are not usually raw, but are from cows fed organically grown feed. Organic dairy products are certainly superior to commercial ones, but a combination of raw and organic is optimal, though difficult to find. The availability of raw milk products varies greatly from state to state. (For more information on this important subject, please visit www.RealMilk.com, or see the Resources section).

Emphasize Whole Foods

Fresh, home-cooked, whole foods are always going to be superior to processed or packaged foods, even ones purchased in a natural food store. Packaged foods certainly have convenience value, and it is unrealistic to expect that you will completely stop using them. However, to the degree that you can minimize such foods, you will be rewarded with superior health. There was a phrase that was popular in the early days of the computer industry: "garbage in, garbage out"! This meant that the information that a computer can give you will only be as good as the quality of the data entered into it. The human body is similar: feed it garbage, and it will become garbage. Remember that the food you eat literally becomes the raw material with which your body builds new tissues and repairs old ones. While other factors—such as exercise, stress, and mental attitude—are also important to your overall health, food provides the literal foundation from which your body is built.

Sugar should be avoided, or used only on special celebratory occasions. Sugar is an anti-nutrient, meaning that it takes more from the body than it gives. It has been stripped of all of its vitamins and minerals during the refining process, yet it needs these very substances to be metabolized by the body. Consequently, it has to steal them from the body's own precious reserves, depleting the body in the process. Non-foods like artificial sweeteners, food additives, preservatives, man-made fats, and sodas should be completely shunned. White flour products should only be used occasionally, and caffeine and alcohol should be used in moderation, if at all. Processed meats, including luncheon meats, are among the very worst of the modern foods, and are usually laden with nitrites and other toxic chemical additives. It is processed meats, not wholesome meats from properly raised animals, that have been correctly identified as contributing to heart disease, cancer, and other degenerative conditions.

Food Allergies

Many people suffer from food allergies and food sensitivities, often without knowing it. If you know you are allergic to any food shown on your diet plan, then simply do not eat it. There is no requirement to eat all the foods shown on the Group I and II food lists; these are simply the main foods you should choose from for your daily fare.

Savor Your Food

Finally, it is very important that you enjoy your food—its taste, colors, textures, and aromas. Find ways to prepare food that are esthetically pleasing to you, and try to eat in a calm, relaxed atmosphere, which both increases the enjoyment of the food and your body's ability to digest it. Even the best food in the world will not be properly broken down and assimilated if it is eaten on the run, in a hectic environment, or in a stressful frame of mind. Use meals as a time to slow down. Eat slowly, chew your food thoroughly (which helps initiate the digestive process), breathe deeply, enjoy the companionship of family and friends, and savor and appreciate the bounty of nature.

Menu Planning

Introduction

So far we have looked at the kinds of foods that should optimally be eaten by the Group I and Group II types to achieve and maintain metabolic balance. In this section we will outline suggested meal plans, or menus. Please keep in mind that *these are suggestions only.* Feel free to adapt existing recipes or create new ones that appeal to you, so long as they follow the basic guidelines for your Metabolic Type. You are limited only by your imagination!

The quantity of food eaten at any given meal will vary greatly from individual to individual. Some of you may feel that the amount of food shown in the suggested meal plans is too much, but for others it may seem just right or too little. Let the feedback from your own body be your guide in determining what quantity of food works best in your particular system. As already mentioned, you should eat enough food at each meal to feel comfortably satiated (otherwise you will be hungry all too soon), but you should avoid overeating (characterized by feeling "stuffed," or heavy, or lethargic), as this places an undue strain on all of the organs involved in the digestive process.

Keep in mind that there are good foods that are good for us, but also good foods that are bad for us. There are also inherently bad foods ("junk food") that are bad for all of us, regardless of our Metabolic Type. Dr. Richard Kunin, an eminent orthomolecular physician in San Francisco, has stated that he could find something wrong with *any* food. Accordingly, it behooves us to focus on foods that are optimal for our particular metabolic needs. However, we do not expect people to become rigid and adhere to the suggested food lists 100%. Not only would this be impractical, but it is also important to not always eat the same foods. The items on the list that is appropriate to your Metabolic Type should be seen as the basic day-to-day staples around which to construct your diet; but it is fine to incorporate other healthy foods to lend variety. Just keep in mind that if you stray too far from the suggested list for your Metabolic Type, it will tend to exacerbate your pH imbalance. Try to eat approximately 80% of your foods from the suggested food list.

FIGURE 3-4   Group I Menu Plan

	BREAKFAST	LUNCH	DINNER
Monday	Yogurt (low-fat) Fruit Almonds	Chicken sandwich Green salad	Grilled sole Steamed greens Baked potato
Tuesday	Wheat (or corn) flakes Low-fat milk Fruit	Turkey burger Coleslaw Mixed vegetables	Chicken noodle soup Pasta (marinara sauce) Steamed chard
Wednesday	Poached eggs Whole wheat toast	Tuna salad Clam chowder	Chicken curry Brown rice Cucumber salad
Thursday	Cottage cheese (low-fat) Fruit Almonds	Chicken salad French onion soup	Broiled halibut Brussels sprouts Green salad
Friday	Cream of wheat Fruit	Chicken burrito Chips (baked) & salsa	Leek and potato soup Eggplant parmesan Green salad
Saturday	Whole wheat waffles Fruit Turkey bacon	Egg salad sandwich Vegetable soup	Chicken risotto Steamed kale
Sunday	Soft boiled eggs Chicken sausage Whole wheat toast	Tuna salad Whole wheat crackers	Turkey breast Potatoes Steamed broccoli

SNACKS

The Group I Metabolic Types generally do not require much in the way of snacks. However, if snacks are desired, they should be selected from the same suggested foods as the primary meals. Suggested snacks include:

> Fruit
>
> Almonds
>
> Yogurt or cottage cheese (low-fat)
>
> Whole wheat (or other whole grain) crackers with low-fat cheese or almond butter.

Figure 3-5   Group II Menu Plan

	BREAKFAST	LUNCH	DINNER
Monday	Yogurt (whole milk) Chicken sausage	Bacon & avocado sandwich Chicken soup	Vegetable soup Meatloaf Green beans
Tuesday	Scrambled eggs Turkey bacon	Chicken Caesar salad Lentil soup	Tuna casserole Steamed artichoke Grated carrot salad
Wednesday	Oatmeal Whey powder Banana	Chicken sandwich Carrot and celery sticks Olives	Baked salmon Steamed cauliflower Spinach salad
Thursday	Soft-boiled eggs Bacon Toast (non-wheat)	Greek salad with feta cheese Bean soup	Roast chicken Sautéed mushrooms Asparagus
Friday	Cottage cheese (whole milk) Blueberries Walnuts	Hamburger patty Corn on the cob Kidney bean salad	Cream of asparagus soup Sardines Spinach salad
Saturday	Buckwheat pancakes Molasses Turkey bacon	Lamb chops Steamed spinach or chard Sweet corn	Miso soup Brown rice sushi
Sunday	Avocado & cheese omelet Toast (non-wheat)	Mixed seafood casserole Quinoa, millet, or brown rice	Steak Carrots & peas Baked winter squash

SNACKS

The Group II Metabolic Types commonly require snacks between meals, especially in the mid or late afternoon. The snacks should be protein and/or fat based; carbohydrates should not be eaten alone. Suggested snacks include:

> Olives
>
> Half an avocado
>
> Sardines or tuna (dark)
>
> Mixed nuts and seeds
>
> Banana with walnuts
>
> Half an apple with a piece of cheese
>
> Celery or carrot sticks with nut butter
>
> Yogurt or cottage cheese (full fat/whole milk)
>
> Rye or brown rice crackers with avocado, cheese, or nut butter.

There are many tradeoffs we have to make. For example, spinach (a Group II food) is high in oxalic acid, which inhibits the absorption of calcium (which is also a Group II nutrient). When we cook spinach, we neutralize the oxalic acid, thereby preventing it from interfering with calcium assimilation. However, we also know that cooking destroys most, if not all, of the healthful enzymes present in raw foods, and it can change the molecular configuration of other nutrients. Therefore, we advocate eating as many as half of your vegetables raw, especially in warmer weather. However, light cooking can actually help certain nutrients become more bio-available. This includes fibrous vegetables like broccoli and kale, and also tomatoes, which contain a potent antioxidant called lycopene that is much more readily available in cooked than in raw tomatoes. Vegetables should never be overcooked, and should retain their vibrant colors.

Food Combining

There are many different theories concerning food combining, many of which contradict one another. (Food combining, as we are using the term here, refers to whether or not to eat certain foods together at the same meal, and should not be confused with selecting foods according to your Metabolic Type). The need to pay attention to food combinations seems to vary greatly from person to person. We could say, somewhat tongue in cheek, that food combining is important only to the degree that it is important! Some people seem to be able to eat any and all foods at the same time with no problem at all, whereas others suffer digestive distress if they stray even slightly from the simplest of combinations.

In general, fruits should be eaten raw, preferably half an hour before a meal, or an hour or two afterwards, to prevent them from interfering with the digestion of other foods, especially raw vegetables; but many people can comfortably combine fruit with such foods as yogurt, cottage cheese, or nuts. Digesting proteins and starchy carbohydrates at the same meal can sometimes be very challenging for people with weak digestion—even though they have traditionally been eaten together for millennia—as can eating more than one protein food at the same meal (such as "surf and turf"). Proteins and vegetables work very well together for almost all people. Milk (especially if pasteurized and homogenized) is generally best absorbed on an empty stomach, as it can interfere with the digestion of other foods eaten with it. Once again, let your body be your guide. If you find that a particular type of meal is hard for you to digest, experiment with a different combination of elements or ratios at the next meal. It is more important to pay attention to how your body feels than to any predetermined theory of food combining.

Breakfast

EGGS

Preparing meals for a family composed of both Group I and Group II Metabolic Types can be a challenge. However, breakfast is usually the easiest meal to prepare in such cases, partly because it is generally the simplest meal of the day, and partly because eggs are one of the few foods that are an excellent choice for people of *all* Metabolic Types. (See Chapter 6 for more information on eggs.) Eggs are a complete protein food and are jam-packed with a wide range of other useful nutrients. The best way to prepare eggs is to boil or poach them; the next best way is to make scrambled eggs or omelets, cooked slowly over a low heat to avoid damaging both the fatty acids in the eggs and the oils used to fry them. Eggs can also be baked as a separate dish, and are a common ingredient in many baked goods. Although we are describing them as breakfast foods, eggs can be a great addition to any meal and are an excellent way to add protein to the diet. Note, however, that scrambled eggs served in restaurants are often made from powdered eggs, a commercial process that oxidizes or damages the otherwise healthy cholesterol in the eggs, creating substances known as oxysterols that can damage the lining of the arteries.[8] If eating out, be sure to ask for fresh, not powdered eggs.

CEREALS

Cereal grains can also be used by all Metabolic Types, although the Group II individuals need to be careful to avoid wheat. In contrast, wheat is the very best grain for the Group I types, but they can also enjoy the non-wheat grains eaten in the Group II diet. The best way to eat grains at breakfast is as freshly ground whole grain hot cereals (cream of wheat, cream of rice, etc.), or as cooked whole grains (amaranth works especially well this way), or cooked flakes (oatmeal, wheat, rye, or barley). However, be sure to avoid the "instant" forms of oatmeal, which have been unnecessarily processed, and often contain sugar. Standard cold breakfast cereals are usually loaded with refined sugar and are highly processed (using high heat and pressure) in ways that damage their proteins and other nutrients. More acceptable versions made with organic whole grains can be found in any natural food store, but even these often have a high sugar content (albeit from natural sources) and are still often processed using similarly undesirable methods. Such cereals should not be eaten daily by children or adults, but ideally would be seen as occasional "fun foods."

JUICES

Orange and grapefruit juice, and other fruit juices are only acceptable for the Group I types. However, even they should drink juices in moderation, due to their high sugar content. Orange and grapefruit juice preferably should be freshly squeezed. If drunk on an empty stomach, chase it down with some plain water. Fresh vegetable juices may be drunk by members of both groups; however, they still often have a high natural sugar content (especially if carrots are used), and so should only be used in moderation, and diluted or chased with plain water. Individuals with blood sugar problems should avoid them completely.

Lunch

Group I meals should center around carbohydrates (vegetables and whole grains), balanced with adequate protein and small amounts of fats (for example, a turkey or tuna sandwich on sprouted whole wheat bread). However, protein should always take center stage in Group II meals, with carbohydrates and fats in supporting roles. Members of both groups can have sandwiches, soups, or various kinds of salads for lunch, although the Group II types need to ensure that their meal contains sufficient protein, and that their sandwich breads do not contain wheat. (For history buffs: sandwiches were invented by John Montagu, the eighteenth century Earl of Sandwich, who pioneered the idea of having a piece of meat between two slices of bread so he would not have to leave the gaming table for an elaborate meal!). When eating out in restaurants, some compromise may be necessary in terms of the specific foods allowed for each Metabolic Type; but Mexican, French, Italian, Chinese and other oriental foods can usually be fairly easily customized to meet the needs of the two different food groups. If eating in Middle Eastern or Moroccan restaurants or delis, Group II types need to remember that couscous and bulgur should be avoided, as they are forms of wheat. Dinner leftovers can also make excellent lunches, while halving the amount of time needed for food preparation.

Dinner

PROTEINS

Dinner can be the trickiest meal for a metabolically diverse family. However, members of both food groups can eat chicken and turkey (light meat for Group Is, dark meat for Group IIs) and share many different kinds of fish. (The Group I types need to avoid salmon and the other oily fish, but Group II types can eat any kinds of fish.) Pasta, noodles, or whole grains can be the centerpiece of the meal for Group I types, but should only be side dishes for Group II types. Group IIs should only eat pasta and noodles made with non-wheat flour (such as brown rice, quinoa, spelt, or corn); because these are also acceptable to Group Is, they can be shared by members of both groups. When eating grain products of any kind, however, the Group IIs need to be sure to eat sufficient protein to balance out the high carbohydrate content of the grains.

VEGETABLES

Vegetables are best prepared by steaming, light sautéing (using low heat and a little water, along with coconut or olive oil), or baking. Boiling is one of the worst methods because the high heat destroys most of the water-soluble nutrients (such as the B-complex vitamins) and leaches out many of the minerals. This can also happen with steaming if it is overly prolonged; vegetables should be steamed only until their colors turn vibrant and they become tender. Try to avoid cooking vegetables in aluminum saucepans, as some of aluminum can leach into your food. (Aluminum toxicity has been associated with neuro-degenerative diseases, including Alzheimer's.) During the warmer months, many of your vegetables can be eaten raw, which preserves their enzyme content and heat-sensitive nutrients. However, as we have already seen, light cooking does help to make nutrients more available in tomatoes and the more densely fibrous vegetables.

Try to buy vegetables in season whenever possible. Local farmers' markets are a wonderful source of fresh, local, and often organically grown produce. Buy the more perishable vegetables in small quantities that you will be able to use right away, and wash them thoroughly before use. As much as possible, try to stick to the vegetables that are recommended for your group, especially for your daily staples.

Grains

Whole grains (especially wheat, rye, barley, oats, spelt, and kamut) preferably should be soaked overnight before being cooked, to leach out some of their phytates (phytic acid) and enzyme inhibitors. These are substances that interfere with the assimilation of their minerals and proteins, respectively, and which can therefore make it difficult to properly digest these foods. This is even more important for beans, which have much higher levels of these compounds; optimally, the soaking water of beans should be changed a couple of times, then discarded. Adding a tablespoon of liquid whey (the fluid which rises to the top of yogurt containers) or a squeeze of fresh lemon juice to the soaking water can make this process even more effective. Grains should be thoroughly washed before soaking or cooking. This is particularly true of quinoa (pronounced "keen-o-wah"), as it contains a mildly toxic substance on its surface that is intended to repel insects; this turns the washing water a milky white, so be sure to rinse it until the water runs clear.

Some individuals are allergic to specific grains (most commonly wheat or corn) but many others are gluten intolerant, a phenomenon that particularly affects people of Northern European origin, especially those from the British Isles and Scandinavia. Gluten intolerance appears to be genetic in origin, and probably derives from an over-consumption of the gluten grains over the centuries by the affected cultures. Gluten intolerance ranges from a mild irritation of the gastrointestinal tract that may never be identified as such, to full-blown digestive distress. Common symptoms include bloating, heaviness, gas, diarrhea, constipation, fatigue, joint aches, and "brain fog." (Many other food allergies or sensitivities share a similar list of symptoms.) If gluten grains continue to be eaten by such a person, the irritation to the digestive tract can lead to malabsorption, intestinal permeability ("leaky gut syndrome"), and various intestinal and systemic diseases.

Strictly speaking, the problem is not gluten *per se* (which is present, to various degrees, in *all* grains) but a particular type of gluten known as alpha-gliadin. It is widely believed that in sensitive individuals alpha-gliadin promotes an immune response, leading to the creation of antibodies which end up damaging the intestinal mucosa, the cells lining the digestive tract. If individuals are gluten intolerant, they need to avoid not just wheat (which is the grain that contains the most alpha-gliadin) but also rye, oats, barley, triticale (a hybrid of wheat and rye), spelt, and kamut. In severe cases, even the South American "seed grains," amaranth and quinoa (which contain smaller amounts of alpha-gliadin), also need to be avoided, as well as soybeans, which often cross-react in such cases. (Buckwheat, despite its name, is not related to wheat, and does not contain alpha-gliadin). Restrictive though this regimen may be, it rewards those suffering from this particular food sensitivity with greatly improved digestion and overall health. Gluten intolerance can be determined by a simple blood test available through any physician. (For more information, refer to *Breaking the Vicious Cycle* by Elaine Gottschall, listed in the Bibliography).

Soups

Soups can be the main course of a meal or a wonderfully tasty side dish. They range from broth, bouillon, and consommés, to vegetable purées, thick stews, chowders, and bisques. They can be served either hot or cold, and with practically any foods. Soups for the Group I types should use vegetable stock, or chicken and turkey broth with the fat skimmed off, a tomato base, or low-fat milk. The Group II types can use heavy cream, thick meat broth (with the stock preferably prepared from bone as well as meat), and whole cheeses. If you are considering a soup for the main course, it should contain the principal protein for the meal; if used as a side dish, consider what the meal needs to balance out the main course.

Salads

Salads should focus on vegetables specific to your group. Mixed green salads would primarily be for the Group I types (though Group IIs may enjoy them two or three times a week), and spinach salads would be for the Group II types. Most of the standard salad vegetables (radishes, cucumber, tomato, peppers, sprouts, etc.) can be added to a Group I salad; Group II salads can include avocado, carrot, celery, peas, and olives. If the salad is to provide the main course for either lunch or dinner, it should include protein foods appropriate to your food group. Both groups can make use of hard-boiled eggs, while a version of the classic Greek salad (feta cheese, spinach, olives, pine nuts, and/or walnuts) works well for Group II types. Vinaigrettes or olive oil and lemon juice work well for Group I dressings, while creamy dressings—such as blue cheese, or ranch—or olive oil with a dash of wheat-free tamari (traditionally fermented soy sauce) work well for Group II types.

Beverages

WATER

Water is the most neglected of all the beverages, probably because it is unsweetened and unflavored and, until bottled waters caught on a few years ago, unmarketable. However, it is the *only* drink that is absolutely essential to human life. Water is needed for almost every single metabolic function—from energy generation and blood building to joint health and detoxification—and the entire body runs better if it is well lubricated with this remarkable substance. Dehydration is surprisingly common and widely overlooked, even though it plays a critical role in exacerbating many common illnesses and degenerative diseases.

On arising in the morning, drink a couple of glasses of plain water to rehydrate the body after the night's deprivation This water may be heated during colder weather, if desired. Typically, six to eight eight-ounce glasses of plain water should be drunk during the day, primarily between meals, or half an hour or so before eating to help prepare the gastrointestinal tract for food. Other fluids, except herb teas, do not substitute for plain water. Tea, coffee, alcohol, and sodas are dehydrating, due to their chemical makeup, despite their high water content. It *is* possible to drink too much water, however, though this is much less common than drinking too little. Research has shown that elderly people, especially those suffering from hypertension (high blood pressure), should not drink too much water, as it can lead to sharp elevations in their blood pressure. Use common sense and "listen" to your body.

Unfortunately, most tap water is of very dubious quality. The chlorine added to most municipal drinking water is not always successful in controlling bacteria, and chlorine itself brings its own set of problems, including playing havoc with the beneficial flora in the digestive tract. Fluoride, which is used by some water districts, is a known carcinogen, a fact that far outweighs its modest ability to control dental decay.[9] Other contaminants, from agricultural run-off to industrial pollution, frequently find their way into tap water, as do residues of pharmaceutical drugs, including antibiotics and estrogen products. In effect, drinking unfiltered municipal tap water is akin to dosing yourself with the waste products of our industrial society!

Spring waters vary greatly in quality, and many of them contain heavy metals (such as arsenic or aluminum) at questionable levels, as well as organic contaminants. Some bottled waters are simply tap water put in a plastic bottle. (The soft drink companies seem to be most guilty of this.) Therefore, a good quality spring water, or reverse osmosis, filtered, or distilled water is your best bet, although the plastic bottles that these are often sold in can themselves leach toxic chemicals into the water, a process exacerbated by leaving water bottles in the sun. Look for the firmer clear or blue-tinted plastic bottles, and avoid opaque ones, or any that easily crumple. Investing in a good quality home filtration system is probably the most reliable solution to this problem.

Tea and Coffee

Some people are highly sensitive to caffeine in any form, and they should avoid tea and coffee entirely. However, others seem to be capable of handling modest amounts of these beverages. Keep in mind, as mentioned above, that the net effect of these drinks is dehydrating, due to their diuretic properties and their stimulating effects, so be sure to drink extra water if you consume them regularly. Coffee and tea used to be universally frowned upon by the natural foods community, but recent research suggests that they do contain certain health promoting substances. This is especially true of green tea, which is loaded with powerful antioxidants known as catechins, but black tea and even coffee also have some positive attributes. Keep in mind, though, that caffeine is addictive, that it does constrict blood vessels, and also stimulates adrenaline production (leading to its famous "speedy" effects). It is also contraindicated in a wide range of conditions, ranging from PMS to hypertension to diabetes (as it can exacerbate insulin resistance).

If you do drink caffeine beverages, favor green tea over the other forms, though some individuals are also sensitive to the tannins that are concentrated in green and black teas. Also, try to find organically grown products. Coffee, in particular, is one of the most heavily sprayed of all crops, and it is generally grown in third world countries with minimal regulations regarding the use of toxic agricultural chemicals, and which often use the very same dangerous sprays that have been banned in the U.S. Decaffeinated coffee (decaf) is another option; try to find decaf made with the non-toxic water processing method, which yields a superior product. Also consider exploring the wide world of herb teas, which contain flavors to please every palette, while simultaneously conferring various health benefits. If you are new to herb teas, peppermint and chamomile are good places to start.

ALCOHOL

Alcohol, like coffee, is a mixed bag. On the one hand it is addictive and, if used excessively, can have extremely grave health consequences; but, on the other hand, small amounts appear to exert a protective effect, possibly because of the antioxidants found in its raw materials (this is especially true of wine). Wine and beer are generally fine if used in moderation (one drink a day) but spirits should be minimized or avoided. Alcohol should be completely avoided by diabetics or anyone else with blood sugar problems, and minimized by those trying to lose weight.

JUICES AND SODAS

As mentioned above, fruit juice should be used in moderation, and only by Group I types. Both groups can use vegetables juices in moderation (i.e. a few times a week); but even vegetable juice can pack quite a sugar wallop. Juices should be freshly made and unsweetened. Sodas should be completely avoided, both regular and so-called diet sodas They are loaded with artificial ingredients, and sweetened with either huge amounts of sugar (ten or more teaspoons in a can of regular soda!) or with potentially dangerous artificial sweeteners like aspartame, a known nerve toxin. A high intake of aspartame, as well as sugar, can lead to insulin and blood sugar imbalances, increasing the risk of diabetes. Furthermore, the excessively high phosphoric acid content of sodas flushes minerals, including calcium, out of the system. This, in turn, can lead to serious mineral deficiencies, and is a prime contributor to the scourge of osteoporosis. Teenage girls often drink copious amounts of sodas at a time of critical bone building in their lives, thereby setting the stage for serious problems later in life. Sodas have no redeeming value whatsoever, and are the epitome of "junk food"—empty calories devoid of nutritional content.

Morning Energy Cocktail

The Morning Energy Cocktail is an optional, but excellent way to start the day for people of all Metabolic Types. It should be modified according to one's diet group, as indicated in Figure 3-6. Drink it with, or in place of, breakfast.

There are three main purposes of this drink:

- ∾ To act as a bowel cleanser and improve transit time
- ∾ To help maintain optimal venous blood pH balance
- ∾ To help maintain higher energy over a longer period of time

Figure 3-6   Morning Energy Cocktail

	Group I *Slow Oxidizers* *Sympathetics*	Group II *Fast Oxidizers* *Parasympathetics*
One cup of milk (cow/goat/almond/rice/ soy milk)	low fat	regular/whole milk
One banana	ripe	firm (with green tips)
Protein powder (whey or rice)	1 scoop	1–2 scoops
Psyllium husks (or flax meal)	1–2 tablespoons	1–2 tablespoons
Essential Balance Oil (Omega Nutrition)	1 tablespoon	1–2 tablespoons
Optional		
Lecithin granules	½–1 tablespoon	1 tablespoon
Brewers' yeast	1 tablespoon	1 tablespoon
Carob powder	½–1 tablespoon	½–1 tablespoon
Blackstrap molasses	½ teaspoon	¼ teaspoon
Ice cubes (purified water)	as desired	as desired

Follow the recommendations above for your diet group. Mix the ingredients in a blender, and take along with your morning supplements.

Psyllium ("silly-um") husks, which are a form of fiber, act as an excellent bowel cleanser, but, for some people, two tablespoons might be too much. If you have any negative reaction to this cocktail, use one tablespoon only; or use one to two tablespoons of flax meal (made from freshly ground seeds) instead. Be sure to drink plenty of water later in the morning, otherwise the fiber itself may be constipating, the opposite effect than desired. Observe your stools. They should be soft, long, and should sink. Two or more bowel movements a day is ideal. Welcome to the Stool Watchers Club of America!

FINE-TUNING YOUR DIET

There are two main issues concerning food consumption: quality (or what kinds of food to eat) and quantity (how much to eat, and in what ratios). Knowing your correct Metabolic Type addresses the issue of quality, or what kinds of food an individual should eat; the following section addresses quantity, including the approximate ratios of macronutrients each Metabolic Type should eat.

These ratios are shown as percentages of calories, not of volume. Carbohydrates and proteins yield four calories per gram, and fats yield nine calories per gram. Most protein foods contain fats, so a significant amount of the fat content in the diet will be ingested in your protein foods rather than added separately. Therefore, it is more important in practice to pay attention to the ratio between proteins and carbohydrates, rather than be concerned with the fat ratio.

FIGURE 3-7   **Macronutrient Ratios**

MACRONUTRIENTS	GROUP I *Slow Oxidizers* *Sympathetics*	GROUP II *Fast Oxidizers* *Parasympathetics*	GROUP III *Balanced*
Proteins	25%	40%	30–40%
Fats	20–30%	30–40%	20–40%
Carbohydrates	45–55%	20–30%	20–40%

ᖴ These ratios are *guidelines only,* and will vary greatly from individual to individual. Do not get caught up in the mindset of seeing meals as mathematical equations! Experiment to find out what works best for you. Notice how your hunger level, energy, and mood change in the one-to-three hour period following a meal; if there is a worsening in any of these areas, experiment with adjusting the ratios at subsequent meals. The body's own feedback is much more important than any theoretical ratios, including the ones shown in the accompanying table.

ᖴ The ratios and quantity an individual eats will be affected by daily activity and stress levels; stress and heightened activity generally require a greater protein intake.

ᖴ The most important carbohydrates to emphasize are non-starchy vegetables; fruits, grains, and starchy vegetables are secondary (especially for Group II types). Try to eat some of your vegetables raw, especially during the warmer months, to preserve their delicate enzyme content.

ᖴ Group II types do better if they emphasize protein foods with a medium or high purine content. High purine foods include all organ meats (liver, kidneys, etc.), sardines, herring, anchovies, and fish eggs (caviar or roe); medium purine foods include all meats, fish, shellfish, and poultry, as well as lentils, spinach, asparagus, cauliflower, mushrooms, peas, beans, and peanuts.

ᖴ As a general rule, everyone should eat three regular meals a day, with a couple of snacks if needed (primarily for the Group II types). Eating breakfast is important to "jump-start" the metabolism in the morning.

ᖴ Never *overeat* (i.e. eat until "stuffed"), which places a great burden on the entire digestive process; but do not *undereat* either, which deprives the body of sufficient nutrient intake; rather, eat until comfortably satiated. Overeating and food cravings are more likely to occur if a person is eating foods wrong for their Metabolic Type.

ᖴ If you feel lethargic or sleepy an hour or so after eating a meal, it might mean that you ate too much, or that you lack sufficient hydrochloric acid (HCl) to break down the foods properly in the stomach (a common problem as people get older). If you feel hungry instead of (or in addition to) feeling lethargic, it may mean that you ate too many carbohydrates at the previous meal, in response to which the pancreas has released so much insulin that it has "crashed" your blood sugar. Try adjusting the nutrient ratios at future meals to lower your intake of carbohydrates, especially starches.

∾ As already mentioned, if you have a known allergy or sensitivity to any food listed on the Group I and Group II Foods list, then either avoid or minimize the use of that particular food. An allergy should supersede the use of a food otherwise suggested for your Metabolic Type. Foods listed on the Group I and Group II Foods list are suggested foods only; it is not required that an individual eat all of these foods.

Balanced Types and the Group III Diet

The Group III diet comes into play when an individual arrives at, or close to, the optimum blood pH. In other words, it is recommended to individuals who are more or less metabolically balanced, with a normal blood pH and an improved feeling of well-being. There is nothing mysterious about this; it is simply what we strive to obtain for all our clients. Both Bill Wolcott[10] and Dr. Rudolf Wiley[11] categorize this person as a Mixed Type. Dr. George Watson[12] used the term Sub-Oxidizer, in the context of the Oxidative system, and Dr. William Donald Kelley has over a dozen intermediate groups between Sympathetic and Parasympathetic in the Autonomic system.[13] It is my feeling that we are all basically talking about the same thing.

A brief point of clarification is needed. After we have metabolically typed individuals as belonging to Group I (Slow Oxidizers or Sympathetics) or Group II (Fast Oxidizers or Parasympathetics), we proceed to optimize their blood pH through targeted foods and supplements. In other words, we use nutrients as the driving force to move them out of an overly acid or overly alkaline condition. There is, however, a wide range within each Metabolic Type; an individual may be only slightly acid or alkaline, or they may be extremely acid or alkaline. The more extreme individuals, at either end of the pH spectrum, are the ones who are more likely to exhibit pronounced symptoms of imbalance or outright disease. Because the ideal blood pH is mildly alkaline (7.46 is 0.46 on the alkaline side of 7.0, the neutral point on the pH scale), many authors claim that an overly acid condition sets the stage for disease,[14,15] but it is equally true that an overly alkaline condition can do exactly the same thing. We use foods and supplements to nudge the blood back toward the optimal pH of 7.46, the ideal acid-alkaline balance. When this occurs many digestive problems, allergies, and other disease symptoms will be alleviated. Often there will also be an enhancement of mood and psychological state, as indicated by Dr. George Watson's original research back in the 1960s. This is what I term a Balanced Type, or Group III, and this is what I strive for with all our clients.

However, sometimes the diet may drive an individual *beyond* the optimal pH range, swinging them from overly acid to overly alkaline, or vice versa. In other words, they appear to have switched temporarily from being a Fast Oxidizer to a Slow Oxidizer, or vice versa; or from being a Sympathetic to a Parasympathetic, or vice versa. In these cases we have overshot our mark, and we have to bring the individual back to the optimal range. The key to success in our protocol is to attain the ideal blood pH. Generally we are correct in our initial Metabolic Typing during the first visit, but sometimes the regime may still need modification at the second follow-up visit one month later. We repeat the exact same testing procedure as on the initial visit, allowing us to observe any changes between the first and second visits. In about 10–15% of cases, we incorrectly type someone on their first visit due to various factors, including mixed metabolic markers, or health or lifestyle issues that can obscure the true Metabolic Type. However, in most of these cases it is usually very obvious at the second visit, after they have been following a controlled diet for a month, what is their true Metabolic Type. Their feeling of well-being has generally not improved, or it may have declined, and their blood pH usually will have worsened (e.g. if they were already acid, it may have become even more acid). For all of these reasons, it is very important that we see clients for a follow-up visit.

There are three categories that our correctly typed clients fall into on their follow-up visits:

1) Significant Improvement

This is our goal, and we strive to obtain this result in all of our clients. We do a complete re-testing on the follow-up visit, and make any minor adjustments if needed. A new appointment is made for these clients three months later, to make certain their blood pH is properly maintained.

2) SOME IMPROVEMENT

These are the clients who have fared well on the program but have not attained their optimal health goals. Most of the time we find improvement in their blood pH, but still they are not in their optimal range. We will then make modifications to their diet and/or supplement regime to encourage the optimization of blood pH. We also review other specific health issues, such as digestive problems, stress, or hormone imbalances. We then schedule the client for another appointment in four to eight weeks.

3) INITIAL IMPROVEMENT FOLLOWED BY
A DECLINE IN WELL-BEING

These are the clients whom we have over-corrected, overshooting their optimal blood pH. The thirty-day check-up will reveal a swing of the blood pH from acid to alkaline, or vice versa. In these cases, our primary modification is dietary only; we simply allow in some of the foods from the opposite food group (e.g. if they are on the Group I plan, we suggest that they now incorporate some of the Group II foods). We then recheck them again in thirty days.

I have observed a few anomalies over the years in performing Metabolic Typing in many hundreds of individuals. Some women will have hormonal shifts at different times of their menstrual cycle that can temporarily alter their Metabolic Type. For example, a member of my family is a Slow Oxidizer, requiring the Group I diet and supplements. However on the first day of her menstrual period she craves heavy proteins, so we simply put her on a Group II regime for five days, and then revert back to the usual Group I protocol. I have another client who reverses her Metabolic Type between her menstrual and ovulation cycles. We simply have her make the proper dietary adjustments during that part of the cycle. These phenomena are usually reported by women, who tell us that they feel great for part of the monthly cycle but poorly the rest of the month. We simply test during each part of the cycle to determine the correct diet. Dr. Rudolf Wiley observed that many people undergo mini-changes during the twenty-four-hour day, probably due to circadian and other biorhythm changes.[16] In a rather unusual scenario, one male client needed to eat Group II foods for breakfast, but Group I foods for lunch and dinner. When he told me of his discomfort after breakfast I simply tested him early in the morning and found him to require a Group II regimen at that time. You might think this is a sophisticated diagnostic observation, but actually it is quite straightforward if the practitioner simply listens to their clients and observes the time frame of their discomforts.

A fifty-one-year-old semiprofessional bike racer came to see me. For the last ten years, Don's general health and energy were excellent during the months of March and April. Toward the end of April, however, his energy would diminish and he was not able to ride competitively for the rest of the year. Don sought medical help from all over the United States, and was given gamma globulin injections, hormones, and hyperbaric therapy (a treatment in which the patient spends time inside a specially pressurized oxygen chamber). Specialist after specialist treated him, but with no success. He struggled with this problem for ten years and was about to give up bike racing when he chanced upon a referral to my office. He requested an interview first, as his experience with other doctors had been so unrewarding, and asked very perceptive questions, grilling me on the possibility of any success. Although I could not guarantee success, I did offer him hope that there was a good chance improvement could be obtained through Metabolic Typing. He reluctantly decided to go ahead, and what was accomplished changed his life.

Our tests showed that in March and April of each year, Don's dominant system was Autonomic Sympathetic. However, through his strenuous exercise, he was exhausting his Sympathetic dominance and changing over to the Oxidative system, becoming a Fast Oxidizer. What was required for him at this point was a complete change in diet and supplements. For two months of the year, while Sympathetic dominant, his diet would consist of low purine proteins, low fat, and high complex carbohydrates. During the remainder of the year he required the completely opposite diet—higher in purine proteins and fats (primarily red meats and oily fish), and lower in complex carbohydrates—to support his Fast Oxidizer dominance. Supplements appropriate to his Metabolic Type changed as well. I had phenomenal success with this client, and he is now able to race all year long.

The Group III Diet

Balanced individuals are still characterized by their fundamental Metabolic Type, and still need to follow the basic principles of their food group. It is simply that they can be more liberal with their food choices, and can incorporate more of the opposite group's foods without being thrown off balance. Therefore, there is no one balanced diet that fits everyone, and, for this reason, we have no set Group III diet plan for our Balanced Types.

Balanced Group I Types

These individuals should still primarily select lighter proteins and lower fat foods, and should include plenty of complex (i.e. unrefined) carbohydrates in their diet. However, they are free to incorporate the vegetables that were previously avoided or minimized, such as avocado, asparagus, carrots, cauliflower, and spinach. Also, more of the richer protein and fattier foods (red meat, salmon, and other oily fish, butter and other whole milk products) may be eaten, if desired. However, too many of the richer foods may throw them out of balance again, and attention should be paid to any signs of imbalance in the body. If need be, they should revert to the original Group I diet until they once again feel more balanced.

Balanced Group II Types

These individuals should still primarily orient their diet around the richer, fattier proteins, with complex carbohydrates in more of a supporting role. However, they are also free to incorporate the vegetables that were previously avoided or minimized, such as broccoli, soft squashes, and the range of salad vegetables and leafy greens. Similarly, they can be more liberal in their selection of fruits, but they should still try not to overdo citrus or sweet fruits, as well as potatoes and tomatoes. They may also want to continue to avoid wheat, which is generally the most de-stabilizing food for the Group II types. Once again, they should pay attention to any signs of imbalance, and be prepared to fall back to the regular Group II diet to regain balance.

LECTINS

Lectins are a type of protein also known as glycoproteins, so called because they bind to carbohydrates ("glyco-") on or in the cell membranes in the body. They are mainly of plant origin, though some also occur in animal foods, especially fish. If a given lectin has an affinity for a particular carbohydrate molecule, the bonding of the lectin to the carbohydrate in the cell membrane will disrupt the cell membrane and damage the cell, possibly leading to its death. A large number of these destructive encounters occurring in the gut wall, the arteries, glands, or any organ set the stage for the breakdown of the body's tissues and a cascade of pathological events.

Lectins can also increase the chances of infectious bacteria adhering to the cells lining the gastrointestinal tract (the intestinal mucosa), as well as causing direct damage to the gut wall itself. This can lead to the possibility of an individual developing food sensitivities, excessive intestinal permeability ("leaky gut syndrome"), reduced absorptive capacity (malabsorption), and dysbiosis—disruption of the intestinal flora, the bacteria that normally inhabit our gut. Not only can these effects lead to localized inflammation or infection, but they can also aggravate any ongoing immune reaction. By interacting with blood cells, lectins are able to influence immune response, and even such metabolic functions as insulin secretion and blood sugar balance.

Lectins have profound implications for autoimmune conditions, which are characterized by a hyperactive immune response where the immune system attacks the very tissues of the body that it is supposed to protect. Some lectins bind to the body's own structural cells, thereby inviting attack by the immune system's army of white blood cells. When this involves the cells of the thyroid or the pancreas, there are serious ramifications for thyroiditis (inflammation of the thyroid gland) and Type I (or juvenile onset) diabetes, respectively; and when it involves the joints, it may initiate the development of rheumatoid arthritis. If an individual has a predisposition for lectin bonding from a certain food, the best strategy is simply to avoid that food. For instance, there are numerous case histories of people who can attest to the reversal of arthritic symptoms simply by steering clear of the nightshade group of vegetables (potatoes, tomatoes, eggplant, and peppers).

Lectins are found in certain foods more than in others, and in varying amounts in the same food, depending on climatic conditions and how the food is processed. The major potentially toxic lectins are found in the following food groups: grains (especially wheat and corn), legumes (particularly soybeans and peanuts); dairy products (more so with cows that are fed grains rather than pastured on grass); and nightshades. For many people, these foods are health-promoting, but for people with lectin allergies they can be health-destroying—yet another examples of how one person's food can be another person's poison. It is worth noting that many of these foods are specific to only one of the two diet groups delineated by Metabolic Typing; for example wheat and the nightshade vegetables are Group I foods, whereas most legumes are Group II foods.

The laundry list of symptoms and conditions that may be precipitated or exacerbated by lectins in sensitive individuals include adrenal insufficiency, allergies, arthritis (both rheumatoid and osteo), asthma, atherosclerosis, attention deficit disorder (ADD), autoimmune diseases (thyroiditis, lupus, multiple sclerosis, etc.), blood sugar imbalances, chronic fatigue, dementia (including Alzheimer's disease), diabetes (Type I), fibromyalgia, high blood pressure, hormonal imbalances, irritable and inflammatory bowel syndromes (Crohn's disease, colitis, etc.), lipid abnormalities, and osteoporosis.[17]

The Possible Lectin Reactions table (see Figure 3-8) lists the main lectin foods that have been tested for each of the blood types. Unfortunately, as research into lectins is still in its infancy, there is much disagreement in this area, with very little consensus among researchers. The following list is drawn from various sources where there seemed to be some consistent consensus. With the clients in our clinic, we often will perform a challenge test for some of these foods using the EAV-Dermatron (an electro-acupuncture unit), but other testing methodologies (such as kinesiology or special blood tests) can also be used for this purpose. Much more research is needed before we will have a definitive understanding of the role of lectins in human metabolism, but there certainly appears to be a correlation between lectins and the Metabolic Types.

It should be stressed that people of each of the various blood types *tend* to react to the particular lectins shown on the accompanying table, but, without further specific testing, there is no easy way to tell if any given individual will *actually* react to any or all of these foods. There is some indication that Rh negative types (e.g. A-) might be more inclined to demonstrate adverse reactions than Rh positive types of the same blood group (e.g. A+), while AB Types (which are the rarest of the four main types, and a hybrid of Types A and B) seem to be much more susceptible to a wider range of food reactions than the other types. You may want to consider getting tested for lectin reactions,

FIGURE 3-8   Possible Lectin Reactions *(Based on ABO Blood Types)*

FOODS	BLOOD TYPE A	BLOOD TYPE B	BLOOD TYPE AB	BLOOD TYPE O
PROTEINS				
Fish:				
flounder	X		X	X
halibut	X		X	X
salmon		X	X	
sole	X		X	X
tuna		X	X	
Legumes:				
black-eyed peas		X	X	
lima beans	X		X	
soy	X	X	X	
CARBS				
blackberries	X		X	X
pomegranates		X	X	
string beans	X		X	
FATS				
chocolate		X		X
sesame seeds		X	X	
sunflower seeds		X	X	X

or minimizing or avoiding the lectin-containing foods that have the potential for being troublesome for your particular blood type.

~ Remember that there is no certainty that an individual in any given blood type will react to any or all of these foods; further testing will probably be required to determine lectin sensitivities.

~ Food allergies or sensitivities are also common to other foods not listed above; other potentially allergenic foods include eggs, corn, dairy, citrus, beef, shellfish, nuts, vegetables of the nightshade family (potatoes, tomatoes, eggplant, peppers), and wheat and all other gluten-containing grains (oats, rye, barley).

 Any food can potentially initiate an allergic reaction in sensitive individuals.

SUPPLEMENTS

We have seen how foods affect members of the two dominance systems in different ways. A food that acidifies the Oxidative types (the Fast and Slow Oxidizers) alkalizes the Autonomic types (Sympathetics and Parasympathetics), and *vice versa*. It will probably come as no surprise, then, to find out that the same principle applies to nutritional supplements. The research into the different effects that supplements can have on Metabolic Types dates back to the 1920s and 1930s with the pioneering research of Francis M. Pottenger, M.D., who, as mentioned earlier, was the father of the Autonomic theory of metabolic dominance. Pottenger discovered that the same supplement would have opposite effects in the sympathetic and parasympathetic branches of the nervous system;[18] a substance that stimulated one branch would tend to inhibit the other. This research was later enlarged upon by William Donald Kelley, D.D.S.

Let us use calcium as an example. Calcium is alkaline forming to the Oxidative types. For the Slow Oxidizer, who is already too alkaline, this would be an undesirable effect, as it would further exacerbate their alkaline tendencies. But for the Fast Oxidizer, who is too acid, calcium would tend to counteract their acid tendency by helping to alkalize the blood. Therefore, supplemental calcium would be undesirable for the Slow Oxidizer but desirable for the Fast Oxidizer.

For the Autonomic types, calcium would have the exact opposite effect: it would be acid forming. This would be detrimental to the Sympathetic, who already runs on the acid side, but desirable for the Parasympathetic, who runs on the alkaline side. Therefore, calcium is seen as a Group II supplement, because it is desirable for our two Group II types, Fast Oxidizers and the Parasympathetics. Conversely, it would be contraindicated—except under certain circumstances—for our two Group I types, Slow Oxidizers and Sympathetics.

"But wait a minute," you might be thinking. "We all know that *everyone* needs calcium to build healthy bones." While it is true that everyone does indeed need calcium (and all the other nutrients, for that matter), the Group I types do not need it in the concentrated form that is found in supplements. Assuming they are eating plenty of green vegetables, dairy products, and other whole foods, they should be able to get sufficient calcium for their metabolic needs from their food. If Group I types consume too much supplemental calcium, they are in danger of upsetting the blood pH balance. The body responds to this by leaching other minerals out of the bones to restore the mineral balance in the bloodstream, thereby actually weakening the bones. Therefore, Group I types do better with other minerals that are more specific to their particular metabolic needs.

Let us now look at magnesium. Magnesium was discovered to be acid forming to the Oxidative types. For the Slow Oxidizer, who is overly alkaline, this would be desirable as it would help to counteract their alkaline tendency by helping to acidify the blood. But for the Fast Oxidizer, who is already too acid, magnesium will tend to exacerbate their condition. Therefore, magnesium would be desirable for the Slow Oxidizer but undesirable for the Fast Oxidizer.

For our two Autonomic types, however, magnesium will have the opposite effect—it will be alkalizing. This is desirable for the Sympathetic, who runs on the acid side, but undesirable for the Parasympathetic, who already leans too far in the alkaline direction. Therefore, magnesium is seen as a Group I supplement, because it is desirable for our two Group I types, Slow Oxidizers and Sympathetics. Conversely, it would generally be contraindicated—at least in supplemental form—for our two Group II types, Fast Oxidizers and Parasympathetics.

Supplemental calcium and magnesium are normally considered to be desirable for all of us, and both are indeed vital for the successful execution of hundreds of different physiological processes. However, as we have just seen, they are only desirable in the concentrated forms found in supplements for certain of the Metabolic Types, and not for the others—at least until the individual starts to show signs of regaining metabolic balance.

Magnesium	Calcium
Slow Oxidizers	*Fast Oxidizers*
Sympathetics	*Parasympathetics*

The same logic can be applied to all nutritional supplements (see Figure 3-9). In some cases a particular supplement is only suitable for one of the two groups (Group I *or* Group II), but in other cases different versions of the same nutrient are required by members of both of the two groups. Vitamin C is an example of this. Group I types do fine with plain ascorbic acid, but Group II types require their vitamin C to be chelated (or attached) to mineral carriers, in the form of calcium ascorbate, or mixed mineral ascorbates.

Some people wonder why they need to take supplements at all. After all, should not our food be capable of providing us with all the nutrients we need? In an ideal world, the answer would be yes; but we do not live in such an ideal world. There are three main reasons why we need to take supplements:

∾ The nutritional quality of our foods has been greatly depleted in the last fifty years due to the use of chemical fertilizers, pesticides, herbicides, and fungicides, over-farming and other agribusiness practices. Due to the exhaustion of the soil, foods today contain significantly fewer nutrients than they did fifty or one hundred years ago. Even organically grown foods, which generally contain significantly higher levels of nutrients than their commercial cousins, are often grown on soil that has been depleted by years of over-farming.

∾ We are facing unprecedented levels of pollution from industrial and agricultural sources, as well as from car exhaust and the numerous hidden chemicals found in every home (cleaning agents, paint, fumes from new carpets and furniture, etc.). All of this places an undue stress on our liver and immune system. Supplemental nutrients, including the all-important antioxidants, are needed to help our body adjust to this never-before-encountered threat to its well-being. Add to this the radiation and the numerous electromagnetic frequencies that bombard us daily, not to mention the extra demands placed on our metabolism by the stresses of our fast-paced lives, and it is not hard to see why we need all the nutrient protection we can get.

∾ Many people do not eat the suggested amounts of fresh vegetables and fruits each day. Supplements help somewhat to make up this deficit, although they should never be seen as substitutes for good food, but as supplemental to it.

We routinely recommend three basic supplements to all our clients:

∾ A metabolically balanced multi-vitamin/mineral supplement (such as Personalized Metabolic Nutrition's *Formula One, Two,* or *Three*);

∾ Digestive enzymes (such as Personalized Metabolic Nutrition's *Kristazyme*) to help people break down their foods, a capacity that tends to decline with age;

∾ Omega-3 and omega-6 essential fatty acids. (See Chapter 6 for an in-depth discussion of the many vital roles of essential fatty acids.) We recommend one tablespoon (or 3–4 capsules) daily of a particular product called *Essential Balance Oil* (by Omega Nutrition) to our Group I clients, and two tablespoons (or 6–8 capsules) daily to our Group II clients.

Personalized Metabolic Nutrition's *Formula One* or *Formula Two* are intended to be "driving" formulas to help nudge the Group I and Group II types, respectively, back into balance. Each of these two formulas deliberately excludes most of the nutrients that are found in the other formula. The reason for this is that these nutrients may further tend to exacerbate the individual's imbalance, due to their effects on the blood pH, until the individual is closer to being metabolically balanced. However, it is not our intention to keep someone on these formulas indefinitely. Usually after a few months we will switch a person away from their group-specific multivitamin formula to *Formula Three,* which includes the entire range of vitamins and minerals.

Formula Three not only includes all the primary nutrients, but, in certain cases, it uses two different forms of the same nutrients. For example, vitamin C is desirable for both the Group I and Group II types; but the Group I types need their vitamin C in the form of plain ascorbic acid, whereas the Group II types need it in the form of calcium ascorbate (or mixed mineral ascorbates). *Formula Three* combines both forms of vitamin C, as well as two forms of vitamin A (palmitate and beta carotene) and vitamin B-3 (niacin and niacinamide). Similarly, many of the minerals are chelated (or bonded) to two different amino acid carriers, as some carriers are more suited to one group than the other. Thus, while *Formula Three* superficially resembles many other multivitamins, it is carefully formulated to balance both Group I and Group II nutrients.

Please refer to the accompanying table (Figure 3-9) to see which supplements are recommended for the different Metabolic Types, and to the Resources section for availability of metabolically balanced multivitamin/mineral supplements.

FIGURE 3-9   Supplements

GROUP I *Slow Oxidizers* *Sympathetics*	GROUP II *Fast Oxidizers* *Parasympathetics*
Beta Carotene	
Vitamin A (Fish Oil, Lemon Grass)	Vitamin A (Palmitate)
Vitamin C (Ascorbic Acid)	Vitamin C (Calcium Ascorbate)
Vitamin D-3	
Vitamin K	
Vitamin B-1 (Thiamine)	Choline
Vitamin B-2 (Riboflavin)	Inositol
Vitamin B-3 (Niacin)	Vitamin B-3 (Niacinamide)
Vitamin B-6 (Pyridoxine HCl)	Vitamin B-5 (Pantothenic Acid)
Folic Acid	Vitamin B-12 (Cyanocobalamin)
PABA (Para-Aminobenzoic Acid)	
Biotin	
Magnesium	Calcium
Potassium	Sodium
Manganese	Phosphorous
Copper	Zinc
Iron	Iodine
Chromium	Boron
Vanadium	
L-Histidine	L-Carnitine

Note: the amino acids listed immediately above (preceded by the prefix "L-") are generally used only for therapeutic purposes, whereas the appropriate group of vitamins and minerals are recommended to all individuals. The Personalized Metabolic Nutrition *Formula One* (for the Group I types: Slow Oxidizers and Sympathetics) and Personalized Metabolic Nutrition *Formula Two* (for Group II types: Fast Oxidizers and Parasympathetics) contain the appropriate nutrients in the correct ratios for the different Metabolic Types. Personalized Metabolic Nutrition *Formula Three* contains the full spectrum of vitamins and minerals, and is for Balanced Types, as well as those with special nutritional requirements. *(See Resources for availabillity.)*

CHAPTER 4

Weight Control
and Other Health Issues

WEIGHT CONTROL AND METABOLIC TYPING

Few subjects in the healthcare field are as emotionally charged as an individual's weight. Advertisers and the media constantly bombard us with idealized images of the human body—glamorous slender women and athletic muscular men—blinding us to the fact that, at least for women, these are simply cultural artifacts. Not only are these images *not* universally shared by other cultures, they are even relatively new in our own. It has only been since the mid 1960s, and the rise of the supermodel, that thin has been "in." Before then, female beauty was associated with a full-bodied voluptuous figure (think of movie stars such as Marilyn Monroe or Jayne Mansfield), as it still is today in many other cultures. Combine this shift with the parallel rise in our obsession with youth and youthfulness, and it is easy to see how culturally determined is our worship of the slender body.[1]

At the same time that the thin body was being enshrined as the new icon of beauty, the medical community was putting forward the theory that dietary cholesterol and saturated fat were responsible for the rise in heart disease. Animal fats became the new evil to be minimized at all costs—despite the fact that humans have eaten animal fats throughout their entire history without suffering from the modern epidemic of obesity; despite the fact that traditional cultures were still eating plenty of animal fats well into the twentieth century while maintaining a high level of health;[2] and despite the fact that heart disease was almost unknown one hundred years ago, a heart attack being a medical rarity before the 1920s.[3]

The simple fact that the same three-letter word "fat" is popularly used to indicate both dietary fats (more properly known as lipids) and body fat (more properly known as adipose tissue) further solidified the supposed link between the two in the public's mind. Fat became public enemy number one—despite the glaring fact that the consumption of sugar and other refined carbohydrates had also risen proportionately with the increase in obesity and heart disease, while the consumption of animal fats had remained relatively steady, or even declined.[4] In 1900, the average annual, *per capita* sugar consumption was five pounds; in the year 2000 it has been estimated to be a whopping 150 pounds![5] Add to this the massive increase in the consumption of other refined carbohydrates (from bagels to breakfast cereal, from white bread to pasta) which all break down to the simple sugar glucose in the body, and we can see that the American diet has shifted radically over the last century towards massive sugar overload. Although it is now becoming more widely accepted that it is refined carbohydrates rather than fats which are the main culprits for our expanding waist lines,[6,7,8] the low-fat paradigm still proves to be very tenacious—doubtless, in large part, because of the huge amounts of money to be made from promoting it.

Research findings from the medical community in the last twenty years have also contributed to our national concern over weight, with troubling statistics linking excess weight and obesity with such degenerative conditions as diabetes and heart disease.[9] Fueled by the combined momentum of these cultural and medical influences, the weight loss industry has become a multi-billion dollar concern, with an endless array of weight loss books, dietary programs, and specialty products parading through the market place, each claiming to offer *the* definitive answer to our growing national weight problem. For some individuals, some of these weightloss plans appear to work, at least in the short term, whereas for others the same plan may be useless, or even dangerous to their health. Herein lies an important clue as to how to best approach long-term weight control: *people of different Metabolic Types need to eat different diets to lose weight.*

Weight Loss for the Different Metabolic Types

Due to the constant barrage of propaganda in the media about low-fat diets, it is hard for many to believe that regularly eating animal protein and good quality fats can actually help the Group II types (Fast Oxidizers and Parasympathetics) lose weight; but, for Fast Oxidizers, proteins and fats help slow down the overly rapid rate at which they tend to burn up carbohydrates (which is what the term Fast Oxidizer indicates). If the energy released from these rapidly oxidized carbohydrates is not used up promptly in physical activity, it is stored in the form of body fat. Alternately, some of it may be stored as excess serum cholesterol or triglycerides; thus, paradoxically, a higher protein and fat diet can actually help *reduce* elevated serum cholesterol and triglyceride levels in Fast Oxidizers and Parasympathetics, even though many of their recommended foods contain cholesterol.

Karen is a thirty-eight-year-old woman who was sixty pounds overweight. She had tried many weight loss programs, but nothing seemed to work for her. We determined her to be a Fast Oxidizer, and so, accordingly, we put her on the Group II diet (relatively high in protein and fats, and lower in carbohydrates). After a few weeks, she sent me an enthusiastic e-mail stating how she had lost over ten pounds, and had more energy than she had experienced in years.

Greg was fifty years old and forty-five pounds overweight. He had been staying away from "fattening" foods, such as butter, meats, oils, and dairy products, but was still unable to lose weight. When we metabolically tested him, we found Greg to be a Fast Oxidizer. The foods he had been conscientiously staying away from were the very foods he required to lose weight! On the other hand, the excess carbohydrates he was eating were causing him to gain weight. When he made the appropriate dietary changes—reducing carbohydrates and increasing fats and proteins—he lost seven pounds and 3% body fat in just three weeks. Although his new diet appeared to fly in the face of everything he had been led to believe by the media and the medical establishment concerning a healthy diet, we can see that it was entirely appropriate for his Metabolic Type.

Unlike Fast Oxidizers, with whom they share the Group II food plan, Parasympathetics tend to have sluggish metabolisms, burning up (or oxidizing) carbohydrates too slowly. Because their metabolisms are dominated by the Autonomic rather than the Oxidative system, eating too many carbohydrates will interfere with optimal autonomic nervous system functioning, which can in turn lead to the deposition of excess body fat. However, the same foods that slow down the oxidation rate of the Fast Oxidizers work to stimulate the activity of the more *hyper* sympathetic branch of the autonomic nervous system in Parasympathetics, thereby increasing their metabolic rate, balancing out the way they use energy, and helping to counteract excess fat deposition.

Slow Oxidizers also suffer from a sluggish metabolism, but, unlike Parasympathetics, they need more complex carbohydrates to speed up their particular metabolism. If left to constantly under-perform, a sluggish metabolism will inevitably lead to the deposition of excess body fat. For Slow Oxidizers, who are controlled metabolically by the Oxidative (or energy generating) system, too many proteins and fats tend to further slow down their oxidation rate, while complex carbohydrates add welcome fuel to the fire of oxidation. Remember, we are *not* talking about simple carbohydrates, like sugar and white flour products, which are nutritionally inferior, and are not recommended for *any* of the Metabolic Types; rather, we are talking about complex carbohydrates, such as whole grains and vegetables, including starchy vegetables like potatoes. Complex carbohydrates are made up of long chains of glucose molecules, which are split apart in the digestive process and quickly oxidized to produce energy. Because complex carbs are rich in nutrients, they provide a significantly superior source of energy to the simple carbs (sugar and refined starches) that deplete the body of the nutrients required for their own oxidation. Complex carbs therefore provide a perfect source of energy for Slow Oxidizers to speed up their lagging metabolism, but are generally contraindicated for Fast Oxidizers whose metabolism is already in high gear.

Michael was sixty-five years old and eighty pounds overweight. Because he had been a vegetarian for forty years, it may be difficult for people steeped in the conventional viewpoint to understand how he could possibly have become overweight. But Michael, who was a Slow Oxidizer, had been eating too many oily foods that were further alkalizing his already overly alkaline blood pH. These had the net effect of further slowing down his metabolism. When he changed his diet to foods that were more acid forming for his Metabolic Type, he began to lose weight. On his second appointment three weeks later he had already lost ten pounds.

Sympathetics, who share the same Group I diet as Slow Oxidizers, are prone to nervous system energy imbalances if they eat too much protein and fat. These foods will further stimulate the activity of the sympathetic branch of the autonomic nervous system, when what they actually need is to raise the activity level of the parasympathetic branch. Although the sympathetic processes do speed up the metabolism, more energy can be produced than is being burned off. Consequently, because excess energy is stored as adipose tissue, it too can lead to the deposition of excess body fat if it gets too far out of balance with the parasympathetic branch. The Group I foods stimulate parasympathetic activity, balancing out the excesses of sympathetic over-stimulation, allowing the Sympathetic types to process energy more evenly and efficiently. While Sympathetics are less prone to weight gain than some of the other types, due to their naturally fast metabolisms, they can definitely put on weight if their parasympathetic activity is overly depressed.

Roland is a man in his early forties with a stressful job in the telecommunications industry. He spends almost all of his working hours in front of a computer, in an environment fueled by caffeine, sugar, and "junk food" of all kinds. Accordingly, Roland had put on a considerable amount of extra weight when he first came in to see us, weighing in at 275 pounds with 43% body fat. After typing him as a Sympathetic, we put him on a lower protein and fat diet and steered him away from processed foods. He lost a few pounds, but soon became frustrated when he hit a plateau. We tried several different supplements to shift his metabolism into higher gear, but it was only when he finally overcame his antipathy to exercise that the pounds started to fall away. Roland had a sedentary job, worked long hours, and was under almost constant stress from the demands of his job. It is unrealistic to think that diet alone will suffice in such situations, and, although his new way of eating remains the centerpiece of his weight loss program, it became clear that he needed to become more physically active in order to attain his weight goal. With the addition of a regular exercise routine that combines a cardiovascular workout with weight training, he has currently lost over fifteen pounds and 5% body fat and, although he still has a way to go, he knows that he is definitely on the right track. He has already been rewarded with improved energy levels, not to mention a new optimism about his future health prospects.

As we have seen, people of different Metabolic Types require different foods to lose weight. What will help a person of one Metabolic Type to lose weight can actually add unwanted pounds to another Metabolic Type. This points to the fundamental premise of Metabolic Typing: *there is no one diet that is right for everyone,* including those who wish to lose weight. Eating for your Metabolic Type, therefore, is absolutely imperative for properly managing your weight in the long term. It also explains why some dieters swear by the high protein and fat approach (as advocated by Dr. Robert Atkins and others) while others find success with the numerous lower protein and low-fat diets on the market. As an added bonus, eating according to one's Metabolic Type will also help to curb the food cravings that often accompany and contribute to weight gain.

Please note that we are *not* recommending a crash diet program, but a food plan intended to be maintained over the long haul. Rapid weight loss (more than two pounds per week) can be very hard on the body, as the excess body fat that is being shed, along with the toxins that tend to be stored in it, can lead to kidney stones and gallstones, as well as to overtaxing the body's detoxification and elimination pathways. We are looking for steady, not rapid weight loss. As the old saying goes: Rome was not built in a day; trying to dismantle it in a day is not a wise strategy.

Additional Factors Affecting Weight Loss

Approximately 60% of overweight individuals will start to see their weight correct itself simply by adjusting their diet. However, eating a metabolically correct diet is not always sufficient on its own to make a person lose unwanted weight. There are many other complicating factors that can interfere with successful weight loss, including hormonal imbalances—such as insulin resistance, estrogen dominance, hypothyroidism, or adrenal insufficiency—numerous prescription medications (including conventional hormone replacement therapy), stress, various pathologies, and certain psychological conditions (such as using excess weight as a buffer against the world). These various avenues will need to be explored in cases where weight loss is difficult to achieve through diet alone.

Many men and women in their late forties or fifties gain weight for no apparent reason. Their diets and lifestyles may not have changed, so why are they gaining weight? The simplest answer to this is the hormonal changes that are taking place. The phenomenon of menopause is widely understood, but andropause (or "male menopause") is not as well known. This is partly because its onset is more gradual, its symptoms less dramatic, and because it has not yet caught the attention of the marketing departments at the pharmaceutical companies. It does, however, account—at least in part—for the infamous potbelly (or "apple shaped") syndrome in men that corresponds to the "pear shaped" menopausal spread seen in many women.

To some degree, these mid-life changes may be inevitable, and they appear to be part of the natural aging process. For example, we all know that the production of estrogen by the ovaries declines in women at menopause; but estrogen is also produced quite effectively by fat cells, while also itself encouraging the deposition of body fat (which partly accounts for why women naturally have a higher ratio of body fat than men). It may well be that part of the reason women tend to put on extra weight in their middle years is to help offset the decline in the production of estrogen by the ovaries, by providing an alternative source in the fat cells.[10] For men, andropause is characterized by a reduction in testosterone levels. Testosterone is famous for its muscle building properties, and it is because men have higher levels of testosterone than women that they tend to have greater muscle mass. As their testosterone levels drop, there is less hormonal input to maintain muscle mass, and so it tends to convert to body fat. Furthermore, this process is often accompanied by a corresponding increase in estrogen levels in men and, as we have already seen, estrogen promotes fat storage.

To successfully cope with these developments, it is often necessary for menopausal women and andropausal men to get a complete laboratory hormonal assay, preferably using saliva samples which can be collected in your own home, and which generally give a more accurate picture of hormone status than blood tests. This would be followed, where appropriate, with a customized hormone replacement program, using the safer natural hormones rather than the more risky synthetic or animal-derived products, which can themselves contribute to weight gain.

Insulin resistance is another prime reason for weight gain, particularly in the middle years, but increasingly and alarmingly, it is even appearing among young people. We will be exploring this topic in greater detail later in this chapter in our discussion of Syndrome X and diabetes; but for now, we should note that the insulin receptors on the surface of the cell membranes become blunted to the effects of insulin after years of overindulging in sugar and refined carbohydrates. Insulin is required to usher glucose into the cells, and once the receptors become swamped and therefore less receptive, insulin levels rise in the bloodstream along with blood sugar. One of the main properties of insulin is to encourage the storage of fat, so excess insulin readily translates into excess body fat.[11] In addition to dietary modification, the best way to improve insulin sensitivity is regular exercise, which "wakes up" the sluggish insulin receptors. Moderate exercise (30–45 minutes, five times a week) should be part of every weight loss program or, for that matter, any healthy lifestyle.

Sub-clinical hypothyroidism is the main reason for many people's weight gain, as well as for the difficulty encountered in losing the extra pounds. The thyroid, a butterfly-shaped endocrine gland located in the throat just below the Adam's apple, is the primary organ in the body that controls our metabolic rate, or the rate at which energy is produced by the cells. We have already seen how a sluggish metabolism (as characterizes Slow Oxidizers and Parasympathetics) can contribute to weight gain, and that this process can be greatly exacerbated by an under-functioning thyroid gland, which can occur in any of the Metabolic Types. Low thyroid function (hypothyroidism) is quite common, especially in women, although it often occurs at a sub-clinical level that does not show up on regular blood tests. If a low thyroid condition is suspected, a full thyroid panel should be performed (including free T3 and T4 levels, reverse T3, and FAMA antibody tests, in addition to the more common TSH test), but often these tests are inconclusive, even though many of the clinical symptoms of low thyroid function may be present. These include cold hands and feet, dry hair or excessive hair loss, fatigue, elevated cholesterol levels, depression, constipation, and weight gain.[12] Low thyroid function is usually treated by pharmaceutical thyroid medications, of which the best known is *Synthroid*. However, various nutritional alternatives can be used, as well as natural thyroid extracts which, unlike the synthetic pharmaceuticals, contain the active form of thyroid hormone, T3, as well as its precursor, T4.

Another factor that can contribute to low thyroid function is mercury toxicity from amalgam ("silver") dental fillings. Although the amount of mercury that leaks from such fillings may be very small, mercury is one of the most toxic substances in the known universe, and even trace amounts released over time can have highly deleterious effects on the body. The thyroid gland is only a few short inches away from the teeth, and it is now thought that many thyroid problems may stem from mercury toxicity.[13] Because the thyroid plays such a key role in overseeing metabolic functions, mercury toxicity could indirectly affect a person's ability to control their weight. While removing mercury fillings is the ultimate solution, it must be performed by an experienced dentist who fully understands the risks involved. (See Chapter 7 for more on dental toxicity.)

Low thyroid function is often secondary to, or caused by, low adrenal function. The adrenal glands, which control numerous physiological functions, including our response to stress, work closely with the thyroid gland in regulating our metabolic rate. The adrenals can be easily weakened by the kinds of sustained, low-level stress we are all exposed to in a fast-paced urban society, an observation that dates back to the groundbreaking work of the Canadian researcher Hans Selye, M.D.[14] Accordingly, adrenal insufficiency is becoming an increasingly common problem. Adrenal insufficiency shares many of the same symptoms as low thyroid function,[15] but also frequently includes dizziness upon standing, and salt craving. It is best assessed through saliva tests of levels of the key adrenal hormones, cortisol and DHEA. Support for over-stressed adrenal glands can be provided by adrenal and other glandular extracts, nutritional supplements (especially vitamin C and the B-vitamin, pantothenic acid), and herbs (such as licorice root and Siberian ginseng).

As we have already mentioned, the single most important thing an individual can do for successful weight management is to eat a diet of foods that are appropriate for their Metabolic Type, as well as engaging in moderate exercise. (Overly strenuous exercise can further weaken the adrenals.) Balancing the metabolism allows the body to most effectively utilize the nutrients from food, leading to a state of homeostasis, or dynamic equilibrium.

Supplements for Weight Loss

Numerous supplements can be found lining the shelves of natural food stores and vitamin shops purporting to help with weight loss. Some of these can be quite effective, while others are useless or even harmful. Several products containing metabolic stimulants, such as caffeine or ephedra, have been heavily hyped in the media. While caffeine and ephedra can indeed speed up the process of thermogenesis (or the burning up of energy), they need to be used cautiously as they can create numerous problems of their own. The more responsible supplement companies will balance these stimulating ingredients with other nutrients that counteract their less desirable properties, but we cannot generally recommend these products unless they are used under the guidance of a nutritionist or healthcare practitioner.

Some supplements that may help, directly or indirectly, with excess weight include:

- **L-tyrosine** (primarily for the Group I Metabolic Types) to speed up the metabolism;
- **L-carnitine** (primarily for the Group II Metabolic Types) to increase the burning of fats as a fuel source;
- **CLA** (conjugated linoleic acid) to facilitate the conversion of body fat into lean body tissue;
- **7-Keto DHEA** to increase thermogenesis and metabolic rate;
- **Thyroid glandulars** (in cases of low thyroid function) to boost the metabolic rate;
- **L-glutamine** and/or **L-glycine** to relieve sugar cravings;
- **5HTP** to address carbohydrate cravings;
- **Lipoic acid** and/or *Gymnema sylvestre* to help regulate blood sugar levels;
- *Garcinia cambogia* extract for improved body mass composition and appetite control.

Keep in mind that none of the above supplements replace the need to properly adjust the diet according to your Metabolic Type. Supplements, as their name implies, should always be seen as secondary (or supplemental) to the diet.

Weight Loss Tips

- Eat according to your Metabolic Type.
- Avoid all sugar, refined starches, partially hydrogenated oils, and other refined vegetable oils (corn, safflower, sunflower, soy, and canola).
- Select fresh, nutritious whole foods, including plenty of vegetables.
- Chew your food thoroughly; avoid eating rapidly; take a deep breath between bites.
- Restrict milk and cheese consumption (but not yogurt and cottage cheese).
- Eat until comfortably satiated, but avoid overeating (feeling "stuffed" or lethargic).

- Eat smaller meals with snacks in-between, which tax the digestive system less than larger meals.
- Do not skip meals (especially breakfast), as this tends to slow down the metabolism.
- Drink 6–8 glasses of water daily.
- Minimize or eliminate alcohol consumption.
- Exercise 30–45 minutes, at least five times a week.
- Do not obsess about your weight; don't weigh yourself more than once a week.
- Accept yourself as you are, even as you apply yourself responsibly to controlling your weight; don't be hard on yourself.
- Investigate any emotional issues that may sabotage your attempts to lose weight.
- If you are taking prescription medications, check with your physician to see if they may be contributing to weight gain.
- Consider checking thyroid and/or adrenal function.

Syndrome X: A Metabolic Typing Perspective

Dr. Gerald Reaven, professor of medicine at Stanford University, noted in 1988 that many individuals were presenting with the phenomenon of insulin resistance, yet could not be classified as Type II diabetics. He named this condition—which was typically accompanied by high triglycerides, low HDL cholesterol, and elevated blood pressure—Syndrome X,[16] a sort of metabolic no-man's-land between normal blood sugar regulation and outright diabetes. Furthermore, these same individuals were at greater risk for developing cardiovascular disease than the general population. Our work with Metabolic Typing—which uses a modified form of the glucose tolerance test to help determine the foods and supplements most appropriate for any given individual—puts us in a unique position to both observe and address this phenomenon.

What *is* insulin resistance? Essentially, it involves release by the pancreas of more insulin than the insulin cell receptors can handle, leading to the condition known as hyperinsulinemia. The receptors are like tiny doorways on the outer surface of the cell membranes that are unlocked by specific bio-chemical "keys." Insulin is a hormone with many important metabolic func-tions, and it has a major impact on our overall endocrine balance. It is essentially an energy delivery and storage hormone. Its two main missions are to deliver glucose into the cells (as glucose cannot get into the cells without it) so that it can be combusted for energy, and to store any excess glucose as adipose (fat) tissue. Fat storage is most likely an evolutionary device that allowed us to store energy so that we could withstand the periods of food scarcity that were com-mon for much of our history. There are several different hormones that can raise the blood sugar levels (such as glucagon, cortisol, and adrenaline), but insulin alone can lower it. From an evolutionary perspective, raising blood sugar—and thereby generating energy—was more important than lowering it. In pre-agrarian times, before cereal grains became a mainstay of the diet, glucose-containing foods were much less common than they are today, so keeping blood sugar levels up was more critical than preventing them from getting too high. Hence the fact that the body has several more tools in its tool kit to raise insulin than to lower it.[17]

Professor Reaven believes that insulin resistance generally develops in response to excess body weight and/or lack of exercise, both of which are results of our increasingly sedentary life styles.[18] Other researchers and clinicians specializing in this area—such as Richard K. Bernstein, M.D. and Ronald Rosedale, M.D.—point the finger at excess carbohydrate intake, especially in the form of sugar and refined starches (bread, pasta, bagels, muffins, chips, cookies, breakfast cereals, etc.).[19,20] These food substances tend to excessively raise blood glucose levels, and in response the pancreas is forced to release more and more insulin to try to clear the glucose from the bloodstream. In fact, more insulin is usually released than is necessary, to increase its chances of succeeding in the vital task of lowering blood sugar levels. Eventually the cell receptors become saturated and simply cannot take in any more insulin—comparable to the way in which a person may "tune out" an annoying sound that will not go away. Accordingly, the receptors start to lose their sensitivity to the insulin "key," and some may even start to shut down, resulting in both glucose *and* insulin accumulating in the bloodstream, a situation which places a great metabolic stress on the body.

Over time, this accumulation has a corrosive effect on the inner walls of the blood vessels, and can lead to elevated triglycerides, lowered HDL cho-

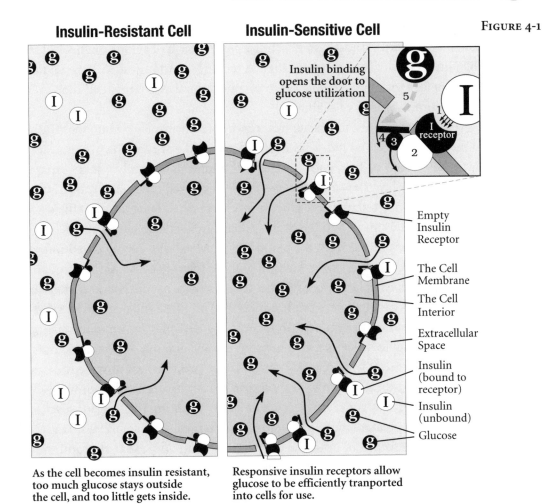

FIGURE 4-1

Insulin-Resistant Cell

Insulin-Sensitive Cell

Insulin binding
opens the door to
glucose utilization

Empty
Insulin
Receptor

The Cell
Membrane

The Cell
Interior

Extracellular
Space

Insulin
(bound to
receptor)

Insulin
(unbound)

Glucose

As the cell becomes insulin resistant,
too much glucose stays outside
the cell, and too little gets inside.

Responsive insulin receptors allow
glucose to be efficiently tranported
into cells for use.

lesterol, and, frequently, high blood pressure—all risk factors for cardio-vascular disease. The clotting factor PAI-1 (plasminogen activator inhibitor 1) may also be elevated, increasing the likelihood of dangerous clotting in the blood, which further intensifies the risk of a heart attack or stroke. Insulin resistance also encourages the development of advanced glycation end products (commonly, and appropriately, abbreviated to AGEs)—mutant hybrid molecules of glucose (or fructose) and protein that are implicated in multiple degenerative disease conditions, as well as in the aging processes itself. Just as hypoglycemia is often a precursor to diabetes, so too is insulin resistance frequently a precursor to cardiovascular disease and accelerated aging.

When Syndrome X develops unchecked in the Group I Metabolic Types, it usually progresses directly to heart disease. When it develops unchecked in the Group II Metabolic Types, it tends to initially manifest as Type II diabetes, before then progressing on to cardiovascular problems and the other classic complications of diabetes.

How does one test for insulin resistance? Measuring the amount of insulin in the blood is one method—fasting insulin should not exceed 12 µIU/mL, and optimally would be below 10 µIU/mL—though this test only offers a "snapshot" and does not show insulin at work. The preferred method of choice is the glucose tolerance test, because glucose levels are directly tied to the efficiency of insulin metabolism, and therefore indicate how effectively insulin is functioning to clear glucose from the bloodstream. Metabolic Typing practitioners use a modified version of the medical glucose tolerance test, as the standard protocol uses such a large dose of glucose (over twice as much as in Metabolic Typing) that it can have very unpleasant effects on those subjected to it. A fasting glucose reading of between 110 and 120 mg/dL indicates impaired fasting glucose; if the glucose levels rise to between 140 and 200 mg/dL after two hours, impaired glucose tolerance is indicated. These two markers provide the primary clinical indicators for what Professor Reaven has termed Syndrome X.[21]

Syndrome X is generally accompanied by a fasting triglyceride level of 200 mg/dL or greater (100 mg/dL, or less, is the most desirable level). Triglycerides are fats found in both the bloodstream and adipose tissue, and they serve as a fuel source for the heart and the muscles. Under normal circumstances, triglycerides are released back into the bloodstream from the fat storage cells when glucose and insulin levels are low (such as first thing in the morning), as a substitute source of energy. Conversely, the release of insulin in response to ingested glucose will normally inhibit the release of triglycerides. In the case of insulin resistance, however, even though there is plenty of glucose in the bloodstream to generate energy, not enough is able to get into the cells because the insulin receptors are overwhelmed. Accordingly, triglycerides continue to be released into the bloodstream to try to make up the energy deficit. Unfortunately, this has the effect of stimulating the liver to synthesize even *more* triglycerides, so that the bloodstream becomes overloaded with them—in addition to the excess glucose and insulin. This process accounts for the excess triglycerides—a prime risk factor for cardiovascular disease—found in people with Syndrome X.

It is estimated that 25–30% of the adult population in the U.S. has Syndrome X,[22] and this goes a long way to explaining the epidemic levels of Type II diabetes and heart disease found in this country. (Several other factors also contribute to high cardiovascular disease rates, as will be discussed later in this chapter).

Two of the most important strategies for both preventing and treating Syndrome X are exercise and weight loss, both of which improve the cells' ability to absorb insulin and, along with it, glucose. The other key area is diet, though disagreement and confusion continues to abound as to what ratio of macronutrients is appropriate. Are Drs. Robert Atkins, Barry Sears, or Dean Ornish correct, each with their own widely varying dietary recommendations?[23,24,25] Professor Reaven does not think so, and he weighs in with his own plan: 45% of calories from carbohydrates; 40% from mostly unsaturated fats; and 15% from proteins.[26] He recommends a food intake of 1,800 calories per day, supplemented with additional calcium. Once again we are looking at a "one-diet-fits-all" approach.

Metabolic Typing takes a different approach. As we have seen, our protocol centers around a modified, or "mini" glucose challenge test. We check the fasting blood glucose level, administer approximately 40 grams of glucose (plus enough cream of tartar to yield one gram of potassium), and then track how effectively the glucose is cleared from the blood over the next ninety-five minutes. Because insulin plays a central role in this process, we can clearly observe the phenomenon of Syndrome X. After successfully performing thousands of such tests over the years, we can categorically state that there is no one diet that is right for everyone. In most cases, balancing the body chemistry metabolically with foods and supplements appropriate to the individual's Metabolic Type will correct glucose dysfunction and lipid abnormalities. In more extreme cases, however, it may be necessary to initiate a special Diabetic Protocol (see Figure 4-2)—emphasizing proteins, good quality fats, and non-starchy carbohydrates—to stabilize blood sugar and triglyceride levels.

Metabolic Typing hinges on the clinical observation that not all people respond the same way to the same foods and nutrients; or, stated differently, that the pH effects of foods in the body are not fixed, or absolute, but rather depend on the Metabolic Type of the person consuming them. Any given food or nutrient will have different pH effects in people of different Metabolic Types. By addressing the individual at the metabolic level, we can maximize the digestion, absorption, and utilization of all foods and nutrients and, by extension, the optimal production and processing of energy.

We will be hearing a lot more about insulin resistance and Syndrome X in the future, as it represents a major breakthrough in the understanding of the development of Type II diabetes and cardiovascular disease. We all owe a debt of gratitude to Professor Reaven for drawing attention to this all too common phenomenon, and we feel that our work with Metabolic Typing has much to offer in both identifying and addressing the detrimental effects of this insidious condition.

DIABETES
❧

Diabetes is the fifth leading cause of death in the US, and its incidence is increasing at an alarming rate, as its precursor condition, Syndrome X, is becoming ever more common. Diabetes is simply the accumulation of too much glucose in the bloodstream (known technically as hyperglycemia), which is often preceded by, and alternates with, hypoglycemia (low blood sugar), as blood sugar levels often fluctuate dramatically in diabetics. This disruption of normal glucose metabolism places a great stress on the entire organism and can lead to a number of serious and potentially fatal complications, including: neuropathy, or nerve damage; retinopathy, or broken blood vessels in the eyes, often leading to blindness; atherosclerosis, or the hardening of the arteries; loss of peripheral circulation, especially in the legs and feet, which, in advanced cases, can lead to gangrene and the amputation of limbs; and kidney failure.

There are two types of diabetes: Type I and Type II. Type I is also referred to as insulin-dependent diabetes mellitus (IDDM), or juvenile-onset diabetes, as it generally makes its appearance in childhood or early adulthood. Type I diabetes stems from irreparable damage to the beta cells of the pancreas, leading to an inability of the body to produce sufficient quantities of insulin to be able to efficiently usher glucose out of the bloodstream and into the cells. Its cause remains somewhat mysterious and may be due to a genetic defect, a virus, or an autoimmune imbalance. Whatever the cause, however, Type I diabetics require insulin injections for the remainder of their lives to be able to adequately clear glucose from the bloodstream, and they must constantly be alert for signs of either too much insulin (insulin shock) or too little (which can lead to a coma). Type I diabetes is a very serious disease, but it only accounts for 5% of all cases of diabetes.

The other 95% of cases are classified as Type II diabetes, also known as non-insulin-dependent diabetes mellitus (NIDDM) or adult-onset diabetes. The term adult-onset refers to the fact that, until relatively recently, Type II diabetes did not typically appear until adulthood, usually not until the middle or later years. This is because it is entirely lifestyle dependent—resulting from consuming excess sugar and refined carbohydrates, and/or a sedentary lifestyle—requiring many years of abuse before its symptoms start to manifest. One of the most tragic aspects of the current "epidemic" of Type II diabetes is that it is now commonly showing up in children, and is closely linked to the disturbing trend towards childhood obesity and the excessive consumption of sugar and refined carbohydrates. One major culprit is soft drinks, which, in their non-diet form, can contain as much as ten teaspoons of sugar per can, and are heavily marketed to children and teenagers. Even diet sodas can contribute to the problem, as *NutraSweet* (aspartame) also initiates an insulin response. Recent research suggests that insulin resistance can even be transmitted from a pregnant women to her unborn child, thereby predisposing the infant to diabetes.[27]

Type II diabetes is the logical (though not inevitable) outcome of insulin resistance and Syndrome X, wherein the ability to effectively transport the glucose into the cells is diminished by overworked or resistant insulin receptors. Therefore, glucose (as well as insulin) starts to accumulate in the bloodstream. While Type II diabetes can usually be controlled without injected insulin, it is sometimes used by medical doctors anyway, in a frequently counterproductive attempt to force the glucose into the cells. In advanced cases of Type II diabetes, insulin may indeed be needed if the pancreas becomes burned out from years of forced overproduction of insulin; but a wiser general strategy is to use newer drugs like *Glucophage* (metformin) or various nutritional or botanical supplements to revive the flagging sensitivity of the cell receptors to insulin.

Type II diabetes is a classic "disease of civilization," almost unknown amongst people eating traditional diets and living in their traditional (non-sedentary) ways. While Type I diabetes is sometimes found among primitive peoples, Type II usually only starts to appear when there is a shift from traditional whole-food diets to the refined and processed foods that characterize the modern western diet. This phenomenon was clearly noted in the 1930s by a Cleveland dentist named Weston A. Price, who traveled the world comparing the dental and overall health of people eating traditional diets to those who had switched to modern foods (e.g. sugar, white flour products, and processed foods). In addition to drastically impaired dental health, Dr. Price found Type II diabetes to commonly occur within a single generation of switching to the modern diet. This and other fascinating observations are chronicled in his classic book, *Nutrition and Physical Degeneration.*[28]

Insulin was first discovered and made available in 1925, over seventy-five years ago. My own first experience with diabetes came when my uncle Henry died from the disease when I was seven years old. Uncle Henry was a loving man who adored his family very much. He had many of his toes amputated because of poor circulation, a common consequence of diabetes, and I remember him with his feet bandaged, using crutches to get around. His death had a big impact on me at such a young age. The discovery of insulin has made diabetes (especially Type I) more manageable, as, before its discovery, it was a death sentence. There is still no cure, but it can be controlled so one can enjoy a good quality of life. However, the best strategy remains prevention, which is easily accomplished through proper diet and moderate exercise.

Around 1969, the first glucose meter (or glucometer) was developed, allowing blood glucose (blood sugar) to be measured from a droplet of blood obtained from a lancet finger prick. The implications of this invention were phenomenal. It meant that blood glucose measurements could be taken quickly and easily any time of the day or night; better still, patients themselves could use this device. It is mandatory that blood glucose be kept within certain parameters, or the resulting imbalance will inevitably lead to disease if left unchecked. Insulin controls blood sugar in a very dynamic manner. The pancreas (which is located behind the bottom half of the stomach, primarily on the left side) is responsible for manufacturing the hormones insulin and glucagon, as well as the pancreatic enzymes (protease, lipase, and amylase) needed for the digestion of food. The alpha cells of the pancreas secrete glucagon, a hormone that is released whenever the blood sugar drops too low. Glucagon tells the liver and muscles to release their stores of glycogen, a starchy form of glucose stored as an emergency back-up supply. The beta cells of the pancreas secrete insulin, which, as we have already seen, escorts glucose into the cells to be burned up for energy. Its other sugar-regulating function is to transport glucose to the liver and muscle tissue for storage as glycogen, or to fat cells to be stored as adipose tissue. Insulin is secreted in two distinct stages: stage one makes enough available to control small amounts of glucose entering the bloodstream; but when more carbohydrates are ingested, stage two kicks in to manufacture even more insulin, albeit at a slower pace. Between stages one and two, insulin should be able to maintain a fasting blood glucose level between 80–100 mg/dL when the stomach is empty, and up to 140 mg/dL following the ingestion of food. The advent of the glucometer has helped diabetics to chart the ups and downs of their own blood sugar, enabling them to take appropriate corrective action.

As many as 80% of Type II diabetics are overweight, even obese, especially around the waist (technically known as visceral adiposity). The impairment of their ability to properly metabolize carbohydrates is both a cause and consequence of the disease. Note that I specifically said carbohydrates, one of the three categories of macronutrients (along with protein and fat). Carbohydrates are composed of carbon (C), hydrogen (H), and oxygen (O), or CHO, while fats are composed of carbon and hydrogen only (CH). Proteins (CHON) are also composed of carbon, hydrogen, and oxygen, but with the addition of nitrogen (N) and sometimes sulfur (S). These are the basic building materials for tissue growth and repair, as well as for energy production. Because of their shared chemical structures, we can demonstrate the interactions between these components. Fat (CH) cannot be converted to glucose because it lacks oxygen. However, glucose (CHO) can be converted to fat, simply by relinquishing its oxygen molecule. Herein lies the problem of obesity. People who consume too many carbohydrates convert what is not needed for short-term energy and glycogen storage into fat tissue. This problem is exacerbated by a sedentary lifestyle, which requires much less energy than is typically produced by carbohydrates. While an excess of dietary fats (especially refined, overheated, or partially hydrogenated oils) *can* contribute to obesity—particularly in the Group I Metabolic Types—it is the excess carbohydrates readily converting to body fat that are usually the prime culprits.

Protein can be converted into carbohydrates as and when needed, and therefore used as an energy source rather than for its usual functions of tissue building and repair. However, this process (known technically as gluconeogenesis) is slow and inefficient because the proteins are reluctant to sur-render their triple-bonded nitrogen. However, to the degree it does happen, glucose can be produced from proteins, with the potential of further raising blood sugar levels. This explains how the body can produce glucose even when fed a diet that contains few carbohydrates.

I have been involved with blood glucose readings since 1987. The ground-breaking books *Nutrition and Your Mind* by Dr. George Watson and *Biobalance* by Dr. Rudolf Wiley convinced me that blood pH was a more reliable marker than the more changeable urine and saliva pHs. I devised the mod-ified or "mini" glucose tolerance test (or glucose challenge) as a simple method to determine the acidity or alkalinity of the blood. It was George Watson who first observed that the more rapid drops in blood sugar levels seen dur-ing glucose tolerance testing are a sign of relatively acid blood; and, con-versely, that slower drops in blood sugar levels indicate relatively alkaline blood. Before I devised this system for ascertaining the pH tendency of the blood, I had to take a venous blood draw (from the infracubital vein in the arm) and measure it with a plasmometer (plasma meter) a very technique-sensitive process. To gain accurate readings, four blood draws were neces-sary, over a fourteen-hour period, making for a lengthy and invasive process. After doing three hundred of these venous drawings, I concluded that this way of testing was not for the masses! I was able to see very few clients, since the test was inconvenient, uncomfortable, and expensive. The mini-glucose tolerance test only involves a two-hour time frame, and is not as costly, uncomfortable, or technique-sensitive, and I believe it to be more accurate for the purposes of Metabolic Typing. Little did I realize back in 1987 that this mini-glucose tolerance test would later prove itself useful for identifying individuals with a predisposition for Syndrome X or diabetes. The mini-glucose tolerance test that I devised differs from the classic form of this test in the amount of glucose used (approximately 40 grams, as distinct from 100 grams), in the addition of one gram of potassium (in the form of cream of tartar), and in the length of the test, which takes ninety-five minutes, rather than six hours. This makes the mini-glucose tolerance test much less invasive and much easier to tolerate than the conventional test.

As stated earlier, Syndrome X is a precursor to cardiovascular disease and/or Type II diabetes. It is my observation that most people who develop diabetes first display symptoms of hypoglycemia (chronically low blood sugar) which, over time, weakens the body's ability to properly regulate glucose and insulin levels. To correct it requires a Group II diet, higher in proteins and fats, and lower in carbohydrates, especially the starchy carbohydrates that convert rapidly into blood sugar. It is also my observation that people with Syndrome X who do *not* display hypoglycemia beforehand tend to go the cardiovascular route, rather than the diabetic route. Unlike the hypoglycemic individuals, they typically require a Group I diet, which is higher in complex carbohydrates, and lower in fats and proteins. Cardiovascular problems certainly are common in diabetics, but I more frequently see them in non-diabetic Syndrome X individuals, requiring the Group I protocol. A few more years of observation and research will shed more light on this complex subject.

Let me now discuss the sequence of dietary and supplement regimes for addressing blood sugar imbalances (dysglycemia) and Syndrome X. I wish to reiterate that I do not diagnose or treat disease. I see myself as a disease-prevention specialist who treats imbalances through the appropriate application of diet and nutritional supplements, preferably before they even manifest as overt diseases. Anytime I see a client that cannot be treated effectively with nutritional protocols, I refer them back to their physician. All clients who come to our clinic are metabolically typed and checked for secondary imbalances. The diabetic that comes in with a fasting blood sugar of over 110 mg/dL is given only a half-strength glucose drink, and if the fasting blood sugar is 140 they are given only one quarter of the drink. The reason for giving them the glucose challenge at all is to evaluate the degree of their insulin resistance. If, for example, a fasting glucose reading of 150 rises to 250, then 265 during our second and third testing cycles, respectively, before dropping to 175 after the final twenty minutes, I know that this patient still has viable insulin competence, albeit heavily compromised. If, on the other hand, this same client's blood glucose keeps rising to 310 during the fourth testing cycle, then I know that we are dealing with a severely compromised insulin response. The prognosis in this situation might not be as favorable with nutritional supplementation alone.

For more technically minded readers, we will be discussing in detail the actual protocols followed during the mini-glucose tolerance test in the Appendix. (Please refer to Understanding the Testing Protocols of Metabolic Typing.) The four glucose readings which are taken at the beginning, then sequentially in thirty, forty-five, and twenty minute cycles, are then analyzed.

A jump of 30–50 points is expected between the first and second readings, taken thirty minutes apart, as the glucose floods the bloodstream. How quickly or slowly the insulin is then able to clear the glucose from the blood during the next two testing cycles indicates the degree of relative acidity or alkalinity of the blood. A balanced blood sugar profile might look something like 80–120–100–90. Glucose readings of 80–135–100–80 demonstrate rapid clearing of the blood sugar by insulin, indicating that the blood is overly acid. By contrast, a reading of 80–135–125–115 demonstrates a slower insulin action, indicating that the blood is overly alkaline. A tendency to hypo- glycemia is revealed by a strongly acid reading of 75–150–85–60. Syndrome X, however, can be seen in both acid *or* alkaline blood, such as the acid 110–190–100–85, or the alkaline 110–190–175–160. In both cases, the blood sugar exceeds the desirable upper limit of 150, indicating dysglycemia. A read- ing of 140–285–300–265 is frankly diabetic (defined by blood sugar that exceeds 200 mg/dL at any point, and/or by a fasting reading of 140 or above), but the drop on the fourth reading suggests a favorable nutritional progno- sis. However, a reading where the blood sugars continue to climb through- out the testing period (such as 160–285–310–330), suggests that nutrition alone may not be able to effect a favorable outcome. This type of scenario usually requires the prescription medication *Glucophage* (metformin) to help reduce blood sugar levels. (Less commonly it may indicate the need for insulin injections, if the condition is sufficiently advanced to have burned out the pancreatic beta cells).

Hyperglycemic conditions tend to give us skewed acid/alkaline readings, as the high blood sugars fall outside the normal reference ranges that we use to calculate the pH tendency. However, we can still use these readings at least to indicate a trend towards acidity or alkalinity. The other markers we use (blood pressure, pulse, respiration rate, breath-holding capacity, etc.) are all very valuable for determining Metabolic Type and, therefore, whether Group I or Group II foods are indicated. Syndrome X individuals with cardiovas- cular problems typically require a Group I diet; while Syndrome X individ- uals with diabetic tendencies require a Group II diet; full-blown diabetics require a special Diabetic Protocol (see Figure 4-2). The Group I Syndrome X individuals with cardiovascular problems are usually not obese, while dia- betics generally are.

Note that individuals taking any medications, or with any known health problem, should consult with their physician before implementing a supplement protocol like the ones shown below.

Nutritional Protocol for Syndrome X with Cardiovascular Tendencies

- Group I diet (lower in proteins and fats, higher in complex carbohydrates)
- *Kristazyme* (digestive enzymes; 1 capsule at the beginning of each meal)
- *Formula One* (multivitamins; 6 capsules daily, in divided doses, with food)
- Fish oil (3 capsules daily, with food)
- Chromium (400–1000 mg)
- Lipoic acid (100 milligrams, three times daily)
- CoQ10 (100–500 mg)
- Gymnema sylvestre (900 mg)
- Vitamin C (as ascorbic acid; 2–4 grams)
- Vanadium (1–5 mg)
- Folic acid (800 mcg)
- Biotin (1000–3000 mg)

Nutritional Protocol for Syndrome X with Diabetic Tendencies

- Group II diet
- *Kristazyme* (digestive enzymes; 1 capsule at the beginning of each meal)
- *Formula Two* (multivitamins; 6 daily, in divided doses, with food)
- Fish oil (4–8 capsules daily, with food)
- Lipoic acid (100 mgs, three times daily with food)
- L-carnitine (2–4 grams, in divided doses between meals)
- Vanadium (1–5 mg)
- Gymnema sylvestre (900 mg)
- Vitamin C (as calcium ascorbate; 2–4 grams)
- CoQ10 (100–500 mg)
- Whey protein powder (20 grams)

Nutritional Protocol for Diabetes

(See Figure 4-2.)

Exercise

No nutritional program for Syndrome X or diabetes can be expected to be entirely successful without moderate (but not strenuous) exercise. Exercise

FIGURE 4-2   Diabetic Protocol

PROTEINS			
Meat	**Seafood**	**Dairy**	**Misc. Proteins**
Emphasize lean meats:	*All are OK, including:*	*Use whole milk or low-fat products:*	eggs
beef	crab	yogurt (plain)	beans
lamb	halibut	cottage cheese	lentils
liver/kidneys	herring	soft cheeses	tempeh
pork	lobster		tofu
poultry	mackerel		
wild game	salmon		
	sardines		
	shrimp		
	trout		
	tuna		

Avoid the Following Foods
- All sugar, honey, fructose, maple syrup, and *all* natural & artificial sweeteners; stevia and xylitol are OK.
- Wheat and all refined grain products (wheat bread, pasta, cookies, bagels, muffins, breakfast cereals, etc.).
- All starchy vegetables (potatoes, corn, winter squashes, turnips, etc.), except for the exceptions shown above right.
- All sweet fruits (including oranges), dried fruits, fruit concentrates, except for the exceptions shown above right.
- All fried foods, partially hydrogenated oils, refined oils, margarine, peanut butter, fast foods, processed foods.
- All milk, cream, hard cheeses, ice cream, mayonnaise, commercial salad dressings, ketchup, popcorn, peanuts.
- All alcohol, sodas (diet or regular), and fruit juices.

General Suggestions
- Eat three regular meals per day, with a couple of snacks in-between; never allow yourself to get too hungry.
- Eat protein with every meal and every snack (e.g. celery/apple & almond butter, nuts, cottage cheese, tuna).
- Eat organic meats, eggs, & produce, when possible; unrefined oils; and lots of vegetables (especially greens).

is probably *the single most effective method for improving insulin sensitivity* and clearing excess glucose from the bloodstream. It also helps with weight control, with improved circulation and overall cardiovascular health, and with a general sense of well-being. However, strenuous exercise should be avoided as it places an additional strain on an already taxed system (especially the adrenal glands, which also play a key role in glucose regulation), but moderate exercise cannot be recommended highly enough. Perhaps the best overall exercise for people with Syndrome X or diabetes is walking, preferably

CARBS			FATS
Grains	**Veggies**	**Fruit**	**Oils/Nuts**
Use whole grains sparingly:	*Emphasize non-starchy, including:*	*3 times a week only:*	*All are OK, including:*
3 times a week:	cauliflower	apples (tart)	almond butter
oats	chard	(Granny Smith,	butter
rye bread	green beans	Pippin)	tahini
No restriction:	green salads	blueberries	oils
rye crackers	kale	pears (firm)	(coconut
	mushrooms	(Bosc, D'Anjou)	olive)
	spinach	raspberries	nuts/needs
	2 times a week:	strawberries	(any
	carrots		raw only)
	onions		
	peas		

- ❧ Drink 2 glasses of filtered or purified water on arising; drink at least 8 glasses per day.
- ❧ Use stevia or xylitol as sweeteners; use cinnamon powder liberally (it helps to lowers blood sugar).
- ❧ Use unrefined (gray/beige) sea salt, such as Celtic, Eden, Mediterranean, Real Salt, etc.
- ❧ Exercise moderately, 5–7 times a week for 30–45 minutes (walking, bicycling, swimming, weight training, etc.).

Supplements (listed in approximate order of importance)
Note: be sure to inform your physician about your supplements, as they may affect your treatment plan.

- ❧ PMN *Formula Three* (multivitamin): 6 caps/day
- ❧ *Kristazyme* (digestive enzymes): 1 before each meal
- ❧ Fish Oil (EPA/DHA): 3000–6000 mg/day
- ❧ Chromium: 500–1000 mcg/day
- ❧ Lipoic Acid: 300–600 mg/day
- ❧ CLA (Conjugated Linoleic Acid): 4000 mg/day
- ❧ CoQ10: 100–500 mg/day
- ❧ Vitamin C (calcium ascorbate): 2000–4000 mg/day
- ❧ Vanadyl sulfate: 1–5 mg/day
- ❧ Biotin: 1000–3000 mcg/day
- ❧ Folic acid: 800 mcg–2 mg/day
- ❧ Gingko Biloba: 120–240 mg/day
- ❧ Gymnema sylvestre: 900 mg/day
- ❧ Taurine: 1000–2000 mg/day
- ❧ L-Carnitine: 2–6 gm/day
- ❧ Whey powder: 1 scoop (20 gm)/day

building up to thirty minutes of brisk walking daily. If that is not possible, then any amount of walking—a ten minute stroll on one's lunch break, or around the neighborhood after dinner—is preferable to none at all.

Diabetes, Cancer, and Weight Survey

Over the past few years I had formed the impression that approximately 80% of my diabetic clients were Group II Metabolic Types (Fast Oxidizers and Parasympathetics), while an equal percentage of my clients with cancer were Group I Metabolic Types (Slow Oxidizers and Sympathetics). To test this hypothesis, I instructed my staff to undertake an extensive analysis of approximately 1,450 of our client files from the previous couple of years. The results (which are tabulated in Figure 4-3) indicate that my hunch was fairly accurate. Approximately 72% of our diabetic clients are Group II types, of which the lion's share (50%) are Fast Oxidizers. This supports the observation that diabetes is often preceded by hypoglycemia (low blood sugar), a phenomenon common—in varying degrees—among Fast Oxidizers. Hypoglycemia disrupts normal blood sugar metabolism and, if left unchecked, can easily flip over into hypergylcemia (high blood sugar). Remember that it is the hormone insulin that is responsible for clearing glucose from the blood. If too much insulin has been produced too often over too long a period of time,

FIGURE 4-3	Diabetes, Cancer, and Weight Survey *(Based on an Analysis of 1,450 Clients)*		
DIET GROUPS	**DIABETES**	**CANCER**	**WEIGHT**
GROUP I			
Slow Oxidizers	16%	35%	15%
Sympathetics	12%	43%	25%
Group I Totals	**28%**	**78%**	**40%**
GROUP II			
Fast Oxidizers	50%	19%	47%
Parasympathetics	22%	3%	13%
Group II Totals	**72%**	**22%**	**60%**

insulin resistance develops, as we have explored in detail earlier in this chapter. A primary consequence of insulin resistance is high blood sugar.

Dr. George Watson, the father of the Oxidative system, believed that most diabetics were Slow Oxidizers, because the relatively long period of time it took them to clear glucose from their blood made them vulnerable to a potentially damaging accumulation of glucose in the bloodstream.[29] However, due to the observed connection between hypoglycemia and diabetes, I had long suspected otherwise, and the data bear me out. Only 16% of our diabetic clients were Slow Oxidizers, while a full 50% were Fast Oxidizers. However, even the Group I diabetics need the special Diabetic Protocol that we discussed above, even though it is modeled after the Group II diet. This is because the need to balance their blood sugar has to take precedence over all other considerations. One of the advantages of our testing protocol is that, not only does it allow us to identify individuals with serious blood sugar imbalances, but it also enables us to detect blood sugar issues before they reach this point. This allows us to help them head off such disease conditions before they have a chance to take hold.

Our data survey also confirmed my suspicion about cancer and Metabolic Types. A full 78% of our clients with cancer are Group I Metabolic Types. What surprised me was that more of them are Sympathetics (43%) than Slow Oxidizers (35%). More research is needed to determine if certain types of cancer are more common among the Group I types than among the Group II types. It is very important for readers to understand that *being a Group I type in no way means you are going to get cancer, just as being a Group II type in no way means you are going to become diabetic.* Only a small minority of our client population has *either* one of these diseases. It also remains to be seen if these data would hold up in a nationwide survey, or if they are peculiar to our particular geographical region in Northern California. What it probably does mean, however, is that the Group I and Group II types seem to have a weakness in one or the other of these two areas. We know that most cancers are environmental in origin (an idea we will be exploring later on in the book); however, it seems that the Group I types are more vulnerable to these influences than the Group II types. However, having a vulnerability in a certain area does *not* predetermine a fixed outcome, and it is precisely our intention through Metabolic Typing to prevent such an outcome. By eating the foods appropriate to your Metabolic type, you will significantly reduce the risk of ever developing either disease, and of becoming another statistic. (We will be revisiting this idea later on in this chapter, in the section titled "Do Genes Determine Disease?").

Our survey also looked at weight gain issues. Almost half of all of our overweight clients (47%) were Fast Oxidizers, with the Group II types accounting for 60% of the total. The second highest group were the Sympathetics (25%), while the Group I types in general accounted for 40% of our overweight client population. We discussed earlier how each of the four Metabolic Types are vulnerable to weight gain, each for different metabolic reasons. However, this survey confirmed my observation that Fast Oxidizers are especially prone to this problem. Clearly this correlates with their tendency to develop insulin resistance and diabetes. Please keep in mind that these figures are a relatively small population sample, and more research will be needed to see how consistently they can be extended to the population in general. However, it does provide additional motivation to get serious about one's diet, and to adopt a food plan that is consistent with one's Metabolic Type.

Homocysteine and Other Cardiovascular Risk Factors

Homocysteine

Any reasonable person can be forgiven for assuming that scientific research is conducted solely for the purpose of discovering new and useful information about the natural world for the benefit of humankind. Unfortunately, the history of science is full of the same benighted forces of ego and power politics, greed and deception that mark other less elevated areas of human endeavor. Lest we think that these forces of scientific ignorance died with Galileo—who paid the ultimate price for daring to question the dominant scientific paradigm of his day—we need only to consider the case of homocysteine.

In the early 1970s the cholesterol theory of heart disease was on the rise. The word "theory" is used deliberately here, as the data supposedly linking cholesterol (both dietary and serum) to heart disease has been so shamelessly manipulated by the medical establishment and the pharmaceutical industry that it has obscured, rather than clarified, precisely what role serum cholesterol does play in cardiovascular disease. (For a full discussion of this important issue, please refer to the following books listed in the Bibliography: *How to Protect Your Heart from Your Doctor* by cardiologist Howard Wayne, M.D.; *The Cholesterol Myths* by Uffe Ravnskov, M.D., Ph.D.; and *Know Your Fats* by lipid researcher Mary Enig, Ph.D.)

During this time, Harvard trained physician Kilmer McCully, M.D., working at Massachusetts General Hospital, discovered a much more significant risk factor for heart disease—homocysteine. Homocysteine is an intermediary amino acid metabolite, meaning that it is a substance produced in the body as a normal but temporary product of protein metabolism. Under normal circumstances homocysteine makes a brief appearance as the amino acid methionine is being converted into another amino acid, cysteine; but under certain circumstances, the conversion process cannot be completed, and levels of homocysteine build up in the cells and spill over into the bloodstream.

These elevated levels of homocysteine wreak havoc in the blood vessels, damaging cells, causing platelet aggregation (clumping of the blood), and unleashing a cascade of dangerous free radicals (unstable molecules that destroy healthy molecules by stealing their electrons). As a result of this assault, plaque starts to form on the inner wall of the arteries. Part of that plaque is cholesterol, which, along with calcium, the body is deploying in an attempt to heal the damaged blood vessels. Blaming cholesterol for the plaque, which can raise the risk of heart attacks and strokes, is like blaming a band-aid for the cut that it is covering. Although you would not know it from all the medical and media propaganda, cholesterol performs many valuable functions in the body, including transporting fat-soluble vitamins to the cells, providing the raw material for all the steroid hormones (estrogen, progesterone, testosterone, DHEA, etc.) as well as vitamin D synthesis, and strengthening the membranes of every cell in the body; it is also a key component of brain and nervous system tissue. Ironically, we have demonized one component of plaque (cholesterol) while deifying another (calcium).

And what is it that allows homocysteine to build up to dangerous levels? In a small percentage of the population there is a genetic defect that impedes the proper conversion of homocysteine, but in the vast majority of cases it is simply a lack of the B-vitamins folic acid, B-6, and/or B-12, or TMG (trimethylglycine, also known as anhydrous betaine). This can be due to dietary insufficiencies (common among people who do not eat plenty of fresh vegetables and other whole foods, or animal protein in the case of B-12), or due to smoking, excess alcohol intake, or oral contraceptives, all of which deplete B-vitamins.

For his revolutionary discovery of what may be the single most common cause of heart disease (a dubious distinction it shares with Syndrome X, in which, as we have seen, insulin resistance leads to elevated triglycerides and depressed HDL cholesterol), Dr. McCully was universally vilified by the scientific community and forced out of his prestigious position at Massachusetts General! Not only did his research dare to challenge the reigning paradigm of the day, but it also threatened the huge profits that the drug companies and food industry were correctly anticipating for their cholesterol-lowering drugs and low-fat foods.

Time and a significant body of research—much of it conducted in the less intellectually partisan climate of Europe—have finally vindicated Dr. McCully, and now, almost thirty years later, homocysteine is being recognized as one of the prime culprits in cardiovascular disease. Unfortunately, due to a lack of pharmaceutical (as distinct from nutritional) options for lowering homocysteine, routine blood panels still do not include a homocysteine test. You will need to specifically request it from your doctor if you wish to assess your own homocysteine levels. Physicians receive most of their ongoing education either directly or indirectly from the pharmaceutical companies, and these companies are not permitted to patent natural substances, like vitamins. Hence they have no financial incentive to promote their use. Homocysteine levels should not exceed 10 μmol/L, and optimally should be lower than 7 μmol/L.

Other Cardiovascular Risk Factors

While we have come to associate heart disease with arteries clogged by plaque, 60–70% of heart attacks occur in arteries that have less than 50% occlusion, or blockage, and 25% occur in arteries that have no plaque at all! Some of the following factors go a long way to explaining this apparent anomaly. Fortunately, all of them are subject to improvement through appropriate diet and supplementation.

Small Particle LDL Cholesterol

As we have seen, there is much misunderstanding about, and exaggeration of, the role of cholesterol in heart disease. In general, the ratio between HDL (high density lipoprotein) cholesterol and total serum cholesterol levels is thought to be more important than the actual cholesterol levels themselves. (An optimal ratio would be 4:1, or lower.) Nevertheless, certain cholesterol fractions may be potentially troublesome for certain individuals. LDL (low density lipoprotein) cholesterol is commonly, if simplisticly, tagged as "bad" cholesterol, because of its tendency to stick to the lining of the arteries, while HDL is labeled "good" because it scrubs away the accumulated LDL. However, both HDL and LDL are actually composed of several different fractions, each with somewhat different properties. HDL is composed of a small particle form that is not nearly as efficient at removing accumulated LDL as its larger form. Unfortunately, a normal blood lipid panel does not distinguish between these forms, so that a person may show an adequate level of HDL, but still be at risk because they have too many small particles and not enough large particle HDL.

Some individuals are also born with a genetic predisposition to over-produce a particular LDL fraction known as small particle LDL (not to be confused with the better known VLDL, or very low density lipoprotein). Small particle LDL is much stickier than the other LDL particles, so it is more prone to form a type of unstable plaque that can easily break off, forming a potentially lethal clot. Individuals with elevated levels of this particular form of LDL run an unusually high risk of heart attacks, often at a relatively early age, even without other risk factors being present, but unfortunately very few doctors are aware of this phenomenon.[30] Furthermore, few labs test for it although the procedure was pioneered by the Berkeley HeartLab (in Alameda, California) in the mid 1990s. (For more information on this phenomenon, see *Eat Fat, Be Healthy* by medical journalist Matthew Bayan, himself a survivor of a small particle LDL heart attack; also, please refer to Resources for availability of expanded cholesterol tests). LDL should predominantly fall under the Pattern A classification to be considered safe (Pattern B is the most atherogenic fraction), and the small particle LDL should be 15% or less of the total LDL.

Lipoprotein(a)

As their name implies, lipoproteins are complexes of lipids (fats) and protein, which, among their other duties, carry cholesterol through the bloodstream. Lipoprotein(a), or Lp(a), closely resembles LDL cholesterol in its structure, but with the addition of apolipoprotein(a), an adhesive protein used to repair damaged tissue, such as artery walls. *Elevated Lp(a) is an independent risk factor for heart disease, carrying a ten times greater risk than elevated LDL,* which, on its own, lacks the sticky properties of apolipoprotein(a). *Elevated Lp(a) can be found even where LDL levels are low.* It frequently accompanies hypothyroid (low thyroid) conditions, making hypothyroidism a potential risk factor for coronary artery disease. Lipoprotein(a) levels should not exceed 40 mg/dL.

Fibrinogen, PAI-1, and C-Reactive Protein

Fibrinogen is a clotting factor in the blood that, if elevated, can contribute to dangerous blockage of the arteries. PAI-1 (plasminogen activator inhibitor 1) is another pro-clotting factor that works by interrupting the body's attempts to break up unwanted blood clots. C-reactive protein is an inflammatory marker that is linked to platelet aggregation, the dangerous clumping of the smallest of the blood cells (platelets, or thrombocytes). If elevated, any of these factors can represent a significant risk factor for cardiovascular disease. Fibrinogen levels should optimally be under 300 mg/dL; PAI-1 levels should not exceed 25 IU/mL; C-reactive protein should be under 2 mg/L.

Magnesium and Vitamin C Deficiency

Magnesium is essential to the proper functioning of the heart. It increases cardiac output, prevents arrhythmia (irregular heart beats), counteracts the buildup of plaque on artery walls, relaxes (or dilates) blood vessels, and reduces stress. Unfortunately, it is commonly deficient in the standard American diet, as most people do not eat enough of its most common food sources (nuts, seeds, whole grains, legumes, and leafy greens). Vitamin C also plays a key role in cardiovascular health by helping to strengthen the walls of the arteries and to prevent the dangerous oxidation of cholesterol and other blood lipids. The great biochemist Linus Pauling believed that vitamin C deficiencies were the leading cause of cardiovascular disease.

Excess Iron

Iron is vital to proper metabolic functioning, but too much iron is damaging to the heart. Iron levels tend to build up in middle-aged and elderly men, and post-menopausal women, the two demographics most prone to heart attacks. Regularly donating blood provides the best protection against excess iron, as iron levels are most easily reduced through blood loss. It is precisely due to such regular blood loss during the menstrual cycle that pre-menopausal women are at the lowest risk for iron overload, and therefore have the lowest incidence of heart disease. Serum iron levels should be under 100 mcg/dL, and are best measured by a serum ferritin test.

Low Testosterone

Although we naturally think of testosterone as a male sex hormone, it carries out a multitude of additional functions in the body. One of these is to build

FIGURE 4-4	Cardiovascular Risk Factors
RISK FACTOR	OPTIMAL RANGE *(the number shown below or lower)*
Homocysteine	7 µmol/L
Triglycerides	100 mg/dL
Small Particle LDL	15% of total LDL (or Pattern/Type A)
Lipoprotein(a)/Lp(a)	40 mg/dL
Fibrinogen	300 mg/dL
PAI-1	25 IU/mL
C-Reactive Protein	2 mg/L
Iron (Serum Ferritin)	100 mcg/dL
Insulin (Fasting)	10 µIU/mL

muscle, and, as the most metabolically active muscle in the body, the heart contains more testosterone receptors than any other muscle. Testosterone levels commonly decline in men as they age, increasing just about every other cardiovascular risk factor described above. Declining testosterone is often accompanied by rising estrogen levels, and, while estrogen appears to play a similar cardio-protective role in women (though not the synthetic forms of estrogen usually used in hormone replacement therapy), it has precisely the opposite effect in men. Though maintaining optimal ratios of testosterone and estrogen cannot be expected to prevent or cure all forms of heart disease, testing levels of these two hormones may be one of the most important cardiovascular preventative measures middle-aged men can take. (For more information on the relationship of testosterone to heart health, refer to *The Testosterone Revolution* by Malcolm Carruthers, M.D., *The Testosterone Syndrome* by Eugene Shippen, M.D., and *Maximize Your Vitality and Potency* by Jonathan Wright, M.D., listed in the Bibliography).

HORMONES AND HORMONE REPLACEMENT THERAPY

Many books and articles have been written on the subject of hormone replacement. Collectively they represent a multitude of conflicting points of views concerning the perceived need (or lack thereof) for hormone replacement, the protocols to be followed, and the preferred methods of administration. The ideas I am presenting here represent a condensation of some of the books and papers I have read on this subject, and a summary of the different protocols I use to address the nutritional problems that result from excessive or deficient hormone levels. This remains a work in progress; although we know much about the complex interactions of the endocrine system and how it affects the body as a whole, there is even more that we do not know. Subsequently, our knowledge has to be seen as provisional and subject to review as new information about this fascinating subject comes to light.

I feel compelled to acknowledge the work of one man whose empirical research and compassionate dedication has significantly advanced our knowledge of the pros and cons of hormone replacement therapy. The books, newsletters, and lectures of John R. Lee, M.D. are an invaluable guide to all who desire greater information on natural progesterone and other hormones. (Please refer to the Bibliography.) He has greatly helped me personally with my own understanding of the role that hormones play in bone demineralization and osteoporosis, and there is no doubt in my mind that natural progesterone (as distinct from synthetic forms, more properly known as progestins) enhances bone growth. As a dentist, I was constantly struggling with the scourge of periodontal disease, the loss of bone around my patients' teeth. The judicious use of progesterone cream, combined with the knowledge of which patients should or should not take supplemental calcium, represents a monumental step forward in solving the riddle of bone demineralization and osteoporosis. I wish to join John Lee's many satisfied patients in offering my most heartfelt appreciation for his groundbreaking work in the area of hormone replacement therapy. Even those who disagree with Dr. Lee's conclusions (and every pioneer inevitably has his critics) have to acknowledge the importance of his voice in the ongoing debate about hormone replacement therapy.

Cholesterol

Take a minute to study the accompanying diagram of the steroid tree (Figure 4-5), so beautifully illustrated by biochemist/nutritionist Steve Fowkes. The tree describes the pathways traveled by the steroid hormones, and the alchemical transmutation of one hormone into another. The roots of this tree are fed exclusively by none other than cholesterol, the fatty substance or sterol (technically, a high molecular weight alcohol) which provides the raw material that distinguishes the steroid hormones from the body's non-steroidal hormones. Steroid hormones are produced both in the gonads (the ovaries in women, and the testes in men) and in the outer layer (or cortex) of the adrenals, walnut-sized glands that sit atop *(ad-)* the kidneys *(renals).* (These natural steroid hormones are not to be confused with the dangerous synthetic steroid hormones often used by athletes to enhance muscle mass and performance). We have all been bombarded with information on the potential dangers of high serum cholesterol, leading to a common but erroneous assumption—held by many medical professionals and lay people alike—that the lower a person's serum cholesterol the better. In fact, low serum cholesterol (defined as 150 mg/dL or less) is extremely undesirable, leading to an

FIGURE 4-5

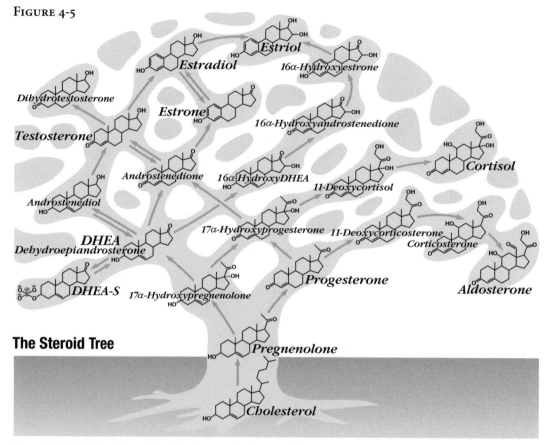

The Steroid Tree

inadequate supply of raw material to manufacture the steroid hormones. This often manifests as low energy or fatigue, depression, and diminished libido. Extremely low serum cholesterol (below 140 mg/dL) is one of the medical warning signs of impending death, and people with cholesterol below 160 mg/dL have a 20% greater chance of developing cancer, and a 40% higher death rate from other causes.[31]

Pregnenolone

The first of the steroid hormones to be produced from cholesterol is pregnenolone, which is the "mother hormone" from which *all* the other steroids are produced. It forms the trunk of our steroid tree, and, when taken supplementally, can be used to elevate mood, enhance cognitive function, and control weight. It is also extremely useful in reestablishing hormonal balance, as we shall see later on. Pregnenolone, fans out to feed all the branches of our steroid tree, each of which is involved in the production of one or more of such key hormones as progesterone, cortisol, DHEA, testosterone, estrogen, and their numerous metabolites. Because they are all nurtured through the same root (cholesterol) and trunk (pregnenolone), *all* these steroid hormones have very similar chemical structures to one another, but the relatively minor structural differences result in major functional differences.

It should be noted that, while we may resort to the common usage of the terms "male" and "female" hormones, there is in reality no such distinction. *Both men and women produce exactly the same hormones*—with women producing the "male" hormone testosterone, and men producing the "female" hormones estrogen and progesterone. The only difference lies in the all-important ratios between them—with men producing significantly more testosterone, and women significantly more estrogen and progesterone. It is these ratios, not the hormones themselves, that define the hormonal differences between men and women.

Progesterone/Aldosterone

Approximately one third of all pregnenolone is converted into progesterone, which occupies the first branch of our steroid tree. The two most important functions of progesterone are: 1) to prepare a woman's uterus for pregnancy; and 2) to maintain a healthy balance with estrogen, so as to protect the body against the potentially harmful effects of its excesses. Copious amounts of progesterone are produced in the ovaries in the second half of the menstrual cycle (the period between ovulation and menstruation, technically known as the secretory or luteal phase), and in the placenta during pregnancy. The elevated levels of progesterone produced in the third trimester of pregnancy enhance the feeling of well-being commonly experienced by expectant mothers at this time. Progesterone production drops precipitously after giving birth, potentially contributing to the postpartum depression that affects some women. This depression can range from a mild and transient case of the "blues" to, occasionally, severe psychosis. As unusually low progesterone levels in general are known to contribute to weight gain, depression, fatigue, loss of libido, headaches, mood swings, and joint pains, it may well also be that the administration of small amounts of natural progesterone might help alleviate postpartum depression.

If we follow the progesterone branch of our steroid tree out to the very end, we will see that some progesterone is also used to make aldosterone. Although this hormone is not generally well known to the public, it plays a vital role in controlling the all-important balance between the electrolytes—especially sodium and potassium—both in the bloodstream and inside and outside the cells. Because of this, it is also directly involved in regulating fluid levels in the body, a function that it shares with the kidneys (which contribute their own hormones, renin and angiotensin, to help in this effort). In cases of adrenal fatigue or insufficiency, aldosterone production tends to drop and, along with it, sodium levels, leading to salt cravings. A person experiencing such craving would do well to add a small amount of salt (¼–1 teaspoon in a glass of drinking water, once or twice a day), both to replenish their sodium levels and to prevent the water they do drink from flushing yet more sodium out of the body.[32]

Cortisol

The next branch of the steroid tree converts pregnenolone into cortisol. Bursts of cortisol released for short periods of time help the body to deal with immediate stressors, by elevating blood glucose and promoting fatty acid mobilization (for increased energy), while decreasing protein synthesis. Cortisol at normal levels also plays a crucial role in regulating thyroid function (since it is required to convert T4 into T3, the active form of thyroid hormone). It assists in controlling allergies, inflammation, and pain, and it helps to wake us up in the morning when its levels are normally at their highest. However, chronic long-term stress (which is common in our fast-paced society) leads to excess cortisol production, at which point cortisol (like excess estrogen) starts to have a catabolic (or tissue damaging) effect, negatively impacting virtually every aspect of our metabolism. Elevated exposure to high levels of cortisol may cause or contribute to high blood pressure (hypertension), reduced glucose tolerance, impaired immune function, insomnia, inflammation, bone loss, hypothyroidism, and other hormonal imbalances—partly by "stealing" more than its fair share of both pregnenolone and progesterone to meet its inflated production needs. Elevated cortisol can also lead to the swamping, and subsequent shutting down of some of the cortisol receptors, which, in turn, can result in increased destruction of brain cells (neurons), accompanied by memory loss. Elevated cortisol (hypercortisolemia) also tends to accompany aging, and it contributes to many of the familiar features that tend to characterize that process.

However, there is only so long that the adrenals can keep producing elevated amounts of cortisol without wearing themselves out. In this scenario, adrenal insufficiency or exhaustion causes cortisol production to plummet, requiring either the medical administration of the prescription drug hydrocortisone to boost cortisol production, or the feeding of more raw material to the adrenals in the form of pregnenolone. (Paradoxically, pregnenolone is also useful in cases of elevated cortisol, to provide more material for the other steroid hormones in compensation for the extra pregnenolone "stolen" to make excess cortisol). Adrenal stress can also result from such major stressors as severe allergies or other illnesses, the death of a loved one, divorce, or the loss of a job. Safe ways to boost cortisol production during such times include administering adrenal glandular extracts, pantothenic acid (and other B-complex vitamins), vitamin C (which is concentrated in the adrenals more than in any other organ in the body), bioflavonoids, adaptogenic herbs (such as Siberian ginseng, ashwaganda, or maca), and whole licorice root extract (glycyrrhizin). Glycyrrhizin ("glissa-rise-in") mimics the action of cortisol in the body, and can benefit a variety of conditions including colds, flu, asthma, allergies, fatigue, and hypoglycemia. However, glycyrrhizin should not be used for a long period of time without supervision, and is contraindicated for people with hypertension, due to its tendency to raise the blood pressure (which is usually depressed in people with adrenal insufficiency).

DHEA

The next major branch on our steroid tree produces DHEA (dehydroepiandrosterone), the most abundant steroid hormone in the body. DHEA—which is sometimes referred to as the "father hormone" due to its key role in the production of the androgens, or "male" hormones—is centrally involved in modulating immune function, balancing blood lipids, counteracting weight gain, and supporting thyroid function. The ratio of DHEA to cortisol is a critical marker of our hormonal health. Cortisol is held in check by DHEA; however, the production of DHEA drops steadily with age, beginning around age twenty-five, and dropping as much as 80–85% by age seventy-five. Cortisol does not decline much (except in cases of adrenal insufficiency); on the contrary, it tends to *increase* with age. A combination of low DHEA and high cortisol can have multiple and often serious adverse effects on our health. Supplementing with DHEA—in amounts ranging from 10–25 mg for women, and 50 mgs or more for men—may have beneficial effects on the heart, immune function, energy levels, libido, and general sense of well-being for middle-aged and elderly people. However, supplemental DHEA is not usually appropriate for younger people, especially pre-menopausal women. It either converts into estrogen (which is already commonly high in pre-menopausal women) or into testosterone, which, in excess, can produce a masculinizing effect in women, such as the deepening of the voice, or the growth of facial hair.

Androstenedione/Androstenediol

DHEA, in turn, nourishes the next two branches of the steroid tree, producing androstenedione ("andro-steen-die-own") and/or androstenediol ("andro-steen-die-ol"). (Androstenedione can also be synthesized from the progesterone metabolite 17-alpha-hydroxy-progesterone). Both of these hormones are anabolic (or tissue building) and androgenic (or masculinizing), and both are readily converted into testosterone, in women as well as men. Supplemental androstenedione and androstenediol offer safe ways to increase testosterone levels in both males and females, especially if taken sublingually (under the tongue) or transdermally (through the skin, in a cream base). By contrast, oral ingestion may produce too rapid a spike in testosterone levels, in a manner that is unnatural to the body. For men, androstendiol may be the preferred form (though, in practice, the two are generally used together) because, unlike androstendione, it cannot be further converted into estrone or estradiol, the two most potent forms of estrogen. This conversion can be prevented by taking the bioflavonoid chrysin (which inhibits the aromatase enzyme responsible for this conversion), just as the conversion of estrone into a benign metabolite (2-hydroxyestrone) can be accomplished by eating cruciferous vegetables (cabbage, broccoli, cauliflower, Brussels sprouts, etc.) several times a week, or by taking special supplements made from them (I3C and DIM).

Testosterone

Testosterone is an anabolic and androgenic steroid hormone that is responsible for the development of the male sex organs, muscles, and facial and body hair. It plays a key role in maintaining human health, strength, and energy, promoting muscle growth, thyroid function, emotional balance, and libido (in women as well as men), while also helping to maintain bone integrity, decrease excess blood clotting, and support overall cardiovascular function in men. (Testosterone is famous for promoting muscle function, and the heart is the most metabolically active of all the muscles; it is loaded with testosterone receptors). Testosterone levels decline with advancing age, manifesting as increased body fat and serum cholesterol, decreased muscle mass, loss of bone density, and diminished endurance and libido. The average male begins to feel a loss of libido and energy between forty and fifty years of age, though this can be minimized or avoided altogether if he properly cares for his body. At the time of this writing I myself am a seventy-seven-year-old male who plays singles' tennis every day, is physically active, and works full-time. In addition, I speak to health groups, conduct weekend seminars once a month for health professionals, and write articles on health issues for various publications. While it is true that my body has aged, and I do not have the energy and libido I had when I was twenty-five years old, I am still able to participate in life to the fullest. My life has been one of moderation, with no excesses. I do not smoke; I drink wine very sparingly, and eat and take supplements appropriate to my Metabolic Type. My own hormone replacement regime consists of 100 mg of pregnenolone and 100 mg of DHEA daily, supplemented by a saw palmetto and beta-sitosterol product to protect the prostate. Perhaps one of the most important aspects of my continued good health is that I look forward to each and every day.

Estrogen

I purposely left estrogen (which, in its various forms, occupies the crown of our steroid tree) for last because it is the most provocative, as well as potentially the most dangerous of the steroids. Estrogen is a primary regulator of the menstrual cycle (most active in the first half of the menstrual cycle, technically known as the proliferative or follicular phase), is crucial to cell division, and is the hormone that produces female characteristics, both in the womb and, later, during puberty. Self-produced (or endogenous) estrogen appears to be protective of the heart and the bones in women, as testosterone is in men, and has positive effects on brain function by stimulating the production of excitatory neurotransmitters (stimulating brain chemicals) known as catecholamines. However, prolonged elevation of estrogen can be quite deleterious and is directly associated with certain cancers. Dr. John Lee describes a syndrome known as estrogen dominance. This occurs when estrogen is unopposed, or insufficiently opposed or counterbalanced by progesterone, producing such adverse effects as PMS (premenstrual syndrome), high blood pressure (hypertension), salt and water retention, abnormal blood clotting, excessive body fat deposition, hypothyroidism, tender breasts, fibrocystic breast disease, ovarian cysts, uterine fibroids, cervical dysplasia, osteoporosis, and a substantially increased risk of breast and endometrial (or uterine) cancer.[33]

Estrogen dominance can occur at any time in a woman's life cycle, both before and after menopause. In fact, it is extremely common for women to exhibit symptoms 10–15 years before menopause, a condition sometimes referred to as pre-menopausal (or perimenopausal) syndrome. In menopausal women, progesterone production often falls to 1%, and estrogen to 50% of their respective pre-menopausal levels. In other words, although we primarily associate menopause with the decline in estrogen production, it is generally preceded and outpaced by a decline in progesterone levels, which can begin as soon as the early thirties. Estrogen is thereby effectively unopposed, creating an overwhelming estrogenic burden on the body. In menopausal and post-menopausal women this may result in the classic menopausal symptoms (hot flashes, night sweats, vaginal atrophy, mood swings, declining libido, etc.), as well accelerating the advance of osteoporosis, and increasing the risk of breast and uterine cancer.

Note that the word estrogen itself does not appear anywhere on our steroid tree. This is because there is no single hormone that bears that name. Estrogen is actually a collective term referring to a group of hormones, of which the most important are estrone (E1), estradiol (E2), and estriol (E3). Estriol is the most benign and protective form of estrogen; estradiol is the most potent and potentially dangerous form; and estrone is somewhere in-between. When we speak of estrogen dominance, and the tumor-promoting effects of estrogen, it is primarily estradiol and estrone (and their various metabolites) to which we are referring.

Hormone Replacement Therapy

Our knowledge about estrogen replacement therapy (ERT) and combined hormone replacement therapy (HRT) has come a long way since the early days of *Premarin* (an estrone-based estrogen replacement derived from the urine of pregnant mares) and *Provera* (a progestin, or synthetic form of progesterone); yet despite the well-documented downside to these two substances, they remain the most prescribed hormones in the world today. Not only do these exogenous (foreign) chemicals *not* behave in the body the same way as their endogenous (self-produced) counterparts do, but estrogen (usually in the form of synthetic estradiol or estrone) is also often prescribed at overly high doses that result in excessive levels of estrogen. Though *Provera* is intended to oppose the estrogen delivered by *Premarin,* it often fails to properly do so, while bringing serious risks of its own. Meanwhile, natural replacement hormones, as well as the phytonutrients that mimic some of the actions of the steroidal hormones, hold out the promise of revolutionizing the practice of HRT.

My own area of expertise is in establishing metabolic balance. I do not diagnose or treat disease; rather I address nutritional imbalances. Oftentimes, hormonal problems exceed the scope of nutritional intervention, and referrals to physicians with a progressive approach to HRT are required; but I do see many women in my practice involved to various degrees with HRT, and I will describe the primary protocols that I use with them. With young women who present with PMS or other symptoms of estrogen dominance, we simply metabolically balance them and use either a high quality natural progesterone cream timed with the monthly cycle, or calcium-D-glucarate, a special form of calcium which helps to clear excess estrogens from the body. (The normal forms of calcium do not have this property.) This usually alleviates problems with excessive bleeding, premenstrual cramps, and mood swings.

For women suffering from menopausal symptoms, the following protocol is recommended:

- ❧ **Stage One:** Use progesterone cream only.
- ❧ **Stage Two:** Use progesterone cream in conjunction with pregnenolone.
- ❧ **Stage Three:** Use progesterone cream, pregnenolone, and 10–25 mg of DHEA. (Note: I never recommend DHEA without having the client first take a salivary hormone panel.)

∾ **Stage Four:** Use all of the above, along with androstenedione, or phytonutrients, as needed.

Sometimes it is necessary to follow all four stages to address the estrogen dominance that manifests as hot flashes and night sweats. We have been most successful with this protocol and recommend it universally.

Hormone Replacement for Men

No discussion of HRT would be complete without addressing hormone replacement for men. As we have discussed earlier, DHEA and testosterone often decline sharply in aging men over time, as does progesterone. The net result is that estrogen and cortisol levels tend to fall out of ratio with testosterone, DHEA, and progesterone. Elevating the levels of these latter three hormones has the potential not only of extending life but of enhancing its quality. We are all programmed to age gracefully, but, because of stressful lifestyles, lack of exercise, inappropriate diet, toxicity and environmental pollution, our longevity and quality of life are compromised. The solution lies in cleaning up our act, becoming metabolically typed so we know which foods to eat and which supplements to take, and making judicious use of natural hormone replacements. *Viagra,* despite its obvious appeal, is not the answer. Although it enhances erectile function in older men, it carries the risk of potentially deadly cardiovascular "side effects," as well as irreversible optic nerve damage.

The following protocol is suggested to enhance male hormonal viability:

∾ **Stage One** (for men aged forty to fifty): Use saw palmetto and beta sitosterol, along with 25 mg of pregnenolone.

∾ **Stage Two** (for men aged fifty to sixty): Increase the pregnenolone to 50 mg; add 25–50 mg of DHEA or 50 mg of androstenedione and/or androstenediol daily; the addition of arginine and choline a few hours before sexual activity may also be helpful, as may the regular use of adaptogenic herbs, such as maca, ginseng, or *Tribulus terrestris.*

∾ **Stage Three** (for men over sixty): Supplement as in stage two, except increase the pregnenolone to 100 mg, and the DHEA to 75–100 mg daily.

Some of the many books written on the topic of hormone replacement therapy are listed in the Bibliography. I cannot emphasize enough the positive impact that lifestyle enhancement and the use of appropriate foods and supplements can have on the health of the endocrine system, and the body as a whole. Even though the world is becoming more and more polluted, we still have the means to protect ourselves from the inside out, and thereby optimize our health and longevity.

NATURAL VERSUS SYNTHETIC HORMONES

Hormones are big business in the US, mainly due to the almost universal practice among medical doctors to routinely prescribe estrogen replacement therapy (ERT) or combined hormone replacement therapy (HRT) to menopausal women. The research on the pros and cons of hormone replacement is often contradictory, but much of the confusion simply stems from a failure to distinguish between the effects of natural and synthetic hormones.

Natural Hormones

The term *natural* is generally understood to refer to a substance directly extracted or derived from a plant, animal, or mineral source, while *synthetic* commonly refers to a substance created in a laboratory. But in the domain of replacement hormones these words take on more specific, if somewhat paradoxical, meanings. *All* commercially available hormones—both those that are referred to as natural *and* those that are referred to as synthetic—are derived from natural sources. Almost all of them come from soybeans or Mexican wild yams (an entirely different botanical species from the edible yams found in our supermarkets, which are, technically speaking, sweet potatoes and not true yams). The one notable exception is *Premarin,* the most commonly prescribed form of estrogen, which is made from yet another natural source—the urine of pregnant female horses (hence the derivation of the name *Premarin,* which is a compression of the words <u>pre</u>gnant <u>ma</u>res' ur<u>ine</u>).

What defines a natural hormone, therefore, is not the source of its raw material, but its molecular configuration. *A natural hormone is defined as one with a molecular configuration that exactly matches the molecular configuration of the corresponding human hormone.* Even natural hormones (other than *Premarin*) have to be altered in the laboratory, because their source materials (soy and Mexican wild yams) do not actually contain any hormones at all. Rather, they contain hormone precursors in the form of sterols, special lipids that have to be structurally modified in the laboratory to convert them into actual steroid hormones. This is analogous to the process whereby the body itself converts cholesterol (which, as its name implies, is also a sterol) into the other steroid hormones, although, in the case of compounds derived from soy and Mexican wild yams, the body is unable to perform this conversion on its own. When the sterols are thus converted in the laboratory into hormones that are identical to those naturally produced in the human body, they are referred to as natural, or, more accurately, *bio-identical* hormones. Almost none of the pharmaceutical hormone products are natural, or bio-identical, by this definition. The one notable exception is *Estrace,* a naturally configured (or conjugated) form of estrogen; unfortunately *Estrace* is made with binders that tend to "glue" or attach it to the body's estrogen receptors so strongly that the body has a difficult time clearing it after it has fulfilled its legitimate function. In other words, it outstays its welcome.

Synthetic Hormones

A synthetic hormone, by contrast, is one where the molecular configuration has been altered in such a way that it no longer exactly matches its corresponding human hormone. The reasons for making such alterations are purely financial, not therapeutic: a strictly natural substance cannot be easily patented, whereas a molecularly altered substance can be, and pharmaceutical companies stand to make much greater profits from compounds that they can patent. By this definition, *Premarin* is considered a synthetic, not a natural hormone product, because several of the forms of estrogen produced by a horse—intended to regulate a much larger mammal with very different metabolic needs than a human being—are significantly different from the human forms of estrogen.

Whenever you change the structure of a substance, you also change its function. Thus, synthetic hormones do not behave the same way in a human body as do natural, or bio-identical, hormones, and they bring with them some potentially very serious risks. This was dramatically underscored in July 2002 when the National Institutes of Health (NIH) abruptly halted the large-scale Women's Health Initiative trial of *Prempro,* a combination of *Premarin* and *Provera,* due to unacceptable increases in the risk of heart disease, stroke, and breast cancer among the trial participants—an act which sent shock waves across the U.S., despite the fact that these "side effects" have been noted in the medical literature for years, and have been strongly warned against by numerous authorities.[34]

Nearly all the beneficial effects ascribed to hormones are true of natural hormones, but not of their synthetic counterparts. For example, synthetic estrogens may effectively relieve hot flashes and other annoying symptoms of menopause, but at a very high price—increasing the risk of breast cancer by at least 20%—while the progestins, the synthetic forms of progesterone (usually medroxy-progesterone acetate, of which the best known brand is *Provera*)—themselves greatly increase the risk of ovarian and uterine cancer. To make matters worse, taking both synthetic estrogen and synthetic progesterone *together* appears to *significantly* increase the risk of cancer over taking them separately—in sharp contrast to how the natural versions of these hormones help to balance one another out. A recent study of more than 46,000 postmenopausal women, conducted under the auspices of the National Cancer Institute, revealed a stunning 40% greater risk of breast cancer among those taking the synthetic forms of *both* hormones.[35] The longer they are used, the greater the risk. It takes four years after a person has stopped taking these hormones for the risk of cancer to subside to normal levels.

Furthermore, while natural estrogen appears to be protective of the heart and natural progesterone to be protective of the bones, there are serious doubts as to whether their synthetic counterparts provide the same protection—despite the fact that they are heavily marketed for *precisely* these purposes. In fact, the published research suggests that synthetic HRT—as distinct from natural hormone replacement—may in fact be quite detrimental to bone density, and may well contribute to, rather than prevent, osteoporosis.[36] Furthermore, recent studies show that women taking synthetic HRT do *not* demonstrate a lower risk of heart disease (which is the leading cause of death in postmenopausal women) than those not on HRT.[37]

To compound the situation, most physicians prescribe HRT without ever first testing hormone levels, nor do they usually perform any follow-up testing. Furthermore, they frequently prescribe hormones (especially estrogen) at doses that far exceed normal physiologic levels. As such, they are essentially experimenting on their trusting patients, rather than tailoring hormone replacement levels to objectively verifiable parameters. In the relatively rare cases that hormones are checked, the older technology of blood serum analysis is usually used, rather than the much more precise saliva testing. The salivary glands, like other tissues in the body, screen out most of the bound hormones (hormones that have become attached to protein molecules, rendering them biologically inactive), and concentrate the free (or unbound) hormones that retain full biological activity. This provides a much more accurate picture of a person's true hormonal status than blood testing, which mixes up both bound and free hormones, often giving the false impression that a person has higher levels of hormones available to them than they actually do.

Unfortunately, the prescription natural hormones (estrogen and testosterone) are not as readily available as synthetic hormones, precisely because they are not marketed by the major pharmaceutical companies, for reasons already mentioned. Instead, they have to be purchased through compounding pharmacies, special pharmacies that—like *all* pharmacies of old—make customized prescriptions from raw materials to fit the precise specifications of the prescribing physician, allowing for adjustments to be made to suit the specific needs of the individual. Compounding pharmacies offer the option of using natural hormones either singly or in combination formulas. For example, while synthetic ERT almost exclusively uses estradiol (or estrone in the case of *Premarin*), which are the two stronger and most potentially dangerous forms of estrogen, the natural versions can be formulated to provide all three forms of estrogen—estriol (E1), estradiol (E2), and estrone (E3)—in ratios that approximate those found in the human body. Alternately, estriol and estradiol may be combined together without estrone, as estrone is synthesized in the body from the other two. When used in this manner, HRT can work with, rather than against the body itself. (Please refer to Resources for information on how you or your physician can contact a compounding pharmacy, as well as for information on saliva testing).

Non-prescription natural hormones (such as progesterone, pregnenolone, and DHEA) are widely available in health food stores, with progesterone usually sold in the form of a transdermal cream. Creams are often the preferred method of delivery for many of the compounded hormone products because only one tenth of the amount necessary for an oral dose is needed to produce the same physiological effect. It is these natural hormones, both prescription and non-prescription, that offer the much touted benefits of HRT, and not their over-hyped and potentially dangerous synthetic analogs.

CHRONIC FATIGUE, FIBROMYALGIA, AND ENVIRONMENTAL ILLNESS

I have taken the liberty of consolidating these three diseases—chronic fatigue syndrome (CFS) or chronic fatigue immune deficiency syndrome (CFIDS), fibromyalgia, and environmental illness—into one category, even though they are three distinct conditions. Again, when we address patients metabolically, we treat the person with the disease, not the disease itself. However, the reason I am discussing these three diseases together is due to the commonalty of many of their symptoms, such as fatigue, depression, mood swings, and headaches. A specific diagnostic description does exist for each of these three, and I would refer anyone seeking more information to the most comprehensive and educational book on these three diseases of which I am aware, *Alternative Medicine* by Burton Goldberg. (Please refer to the Bibliography.)

There are many factors that can contribute to these three disease systems, including the following:

- Infections: by viruses, bacteria, parasites, yeasts (such as candida albicans), and molds;
- Immune dysfunction: autoimmune imbalances, depressed immunity, low lymphocyte (white blood cell) levels;
- Endocrine imbalances: adrenal insufficiency, low thyroid function (hypothyroidism);
- Toxicity: environmental pollutants, agricultural chemicals in our food and water, dental amalgams (mercury fillings), other heavy metals, and pharmaceutical drugs;
- Enzyme deficiencies: both digestive enzymes and the other enzymes that power all of our metabolic processes;
- Allergies and sensitivities: to foods, pollen and other airborne compounds, toxic metals;

∾ Nutritional deficiencies: not only are many people not getting enough of the proper nutrients to sustain health, but they are also eating foods that are inappropriate for them metabolically (remember, there are good foods that are good for us, and there are good foods that are bad for us, as well as foods that are bad for everybody);

∾ Lifestyle issues: stress, psychological/emotional factors.

The number of people suffering from varying degrees of chronic fatigue is staggering, accounting for perhaps as much as 25–30% of the entire population—though a far fewer number suffer from one of these three medically defined conditions. The most common medical approach is to alleviate symptoms through drug therapy, but this neither addresses the cause nor does it offer a cure. As Burton Goldberg points out, it is mainly women who suffer from these conditions, and all three disorders share the dubious distinction of being not well understood by the medical profession.[38]

The most important procedure for these distressed individuals is to determine their Metabolic Type. Once we know which foods and supplements are their allies and, conversely, which create imbalance, our biggest hurdle is surmounted. Following the correct nutritional plan will, in most cases, balance their blood pH over time, allowing for improved digestion, absorption, assimilation, and utilization of macro- and micronutrients. To try to treat a disease system while constantly bombarding the individual with foods and supplements that work against their optimal blood pH is sheer folly. Practitioners who are addressing their patients at a metabolic level are likely to experience a much greater degree of success with *any* disease condition, from cancer to the common cold, even though their main focus will not be the disease itself, but regaining metabolic balance in the body. This is not to say that Metabolic Typing is a magic bullet that makes all diseases vanish overnight, but it does put the body in the best position to deal with whatever health challenges face it.

We may also perform or recommend the following tests:

∾ Checking for secondary metabolic imbalances: anabolic/catabolic, electrolyte stress/electrolyte insufficiency, and acidosis/alkalosis;

∾ Electrodermal (electro-acupuncture) screening: not used as a diagnostic test but to determine organ weakness, and to chart improvements on follow-up visits; it is also helpful for testing allergies;

- Live cell analysis (darkfield microscopy): to obtain a baseline reading on the status of the blood, and to note any anomalies, so we can chart progress on subsequent visits;
- Saliva hormone panel: evaluating cortisol, DHEA, progesterone, testosterone, and estrogen;
- Laboratory blood analysis: lipid panel, liver function, natural killer (NK) cell activity, status of T and B lymphocytes;
- Heavy metal screening.

Chronic fatigue syndrome, fibromyalgia, and environmental illness are complicated, multifactorial diseases, each requiring an individualized approach. However, I cannot emphasize enough the importance of Metabolic Typing as the first and most important step on the road to healing, regardless of how many additional functions and processes need to be evaluated. The whole body must be addressed at the metabolic level, and the individual needs to be prepared to make lifestyle changes. Most important of all is the cultivation of a positive mental attitude.

DO GENES DETERMINE DISEASE?

We live in exciting times for anyone interested in the life sciences. The Human Genome Project has amazed the world with the speed with which it has identified, or "decoded" all of the genes locked within the twenty-three pairs of chromosomes that are collectively known as our genome. These genes contain the blueprint for the structure and functioning of our bodies, and the implications of their decoding for treating disease, understanding the aging process, and, quite possibly, significantly extending human life-span are profound.

However, some caution is also warranted. First of all, the social implications must be considered. For example, will genetic testing be required in the future by insurance companies, and will coverage either be denied or offered at substantially higher rates to people who display the genes associated with particular chronic diseases? And what would be the psychological and social impact on individuals to be informed that they bore the genes associated with cancer or cardiovascular disease? Meanwhile, the pharmaceutical companies are salivating at the prospect of developing a whole new class of drugs that directly target specific genetic predispositions.

This situation points to two closely related concepts that have tended to characterize Western thinking since the rise of the scientific worldview in the last couple of hundred years. The first is reductionism, or the tendency to reduce complex situations to their individual component parts; the second is determinism, or the belief that an outcome is entirely predetermined by its constituent causes. When it comes to our genetic inheritance, we must be cautious neither to reduce all human experience to a genetic model nor to assume that a genetic predisposition equals a predetermined outcome.

These issues are elegantly explored by one of the country's most respected nutritionists and biochemical researchers, Jeffrey Bland, Ph.D., in his book *Genetic Nutritioneering*. Bland argues that genes in and of themselves do not give rise to disease; rather disease results from a complex interaction of environmental or lifestyle factors that alter the expression of the genes in the direction of a specific disease system. Thus, your genotype is modified to express the phenotype (or manifestation) of a particular disease. Stated differently, a genetic predisposition does not imply a predictable result. As Bland puts it: "In terms of your health or disease state as an adult, your phenotype is determined by the way you have treated your genes throughout your life."[39]

Diet, environment, and lifestyle factors, such as stress, play major roles in determining the health of an individual. A recent study performed by the internationally renowned Karolinska Institute in Sweden tracked almost 45,000 pairs of twins to assess the role that genetic heredity plays in the development of cancer. This exhaustive study showed that environmental, not genetic, factors were the primary cause of cancer in upwards of 64% of the cases studied, and as much as 72% in the case of breast cancer.[40] Other studies have suggested that environmental factors are responsible for 80–90% of cancers.

Foremost among these factors are chemical pollutants and toxins, and exposure to radiation (including medical x-rays) and powerful electromagnetic fields. The bad news is that we cannot entirely protect ourselves from these influences, short of lobbying for more stringent environmental controls. The good news is that we can do a lot to protect our internal environment from the negative impact of the external environment. Diet, supplementation, exercise, and stress reduction all play crucial roles in determining how effective the body will be in responding to these environmental challenges. Metabolic Typing can be seen in this context as a powerful way to modify gene expression. As Bland says: "All the genetic messages you need to remake yourself are present in every cell of your body."[41] By feeding our body the foods and supplements appropriate to our particular metabolism, we give our genes the stimuli they need to remake ourselves in the image of optimal health and longevity.

CHAPTER 5

Nutitional Support for Cancer

A New Look At Cancer

As a nutritionist, I do not treat cancer *per se,* or any other disease for that matter. I simply employ the most efficacious nutritional means at my disposal to enhance the ability of the client's own body to heal itself. As there are many different types of cancers, our nutritional recommendations may vary. Some of my clients have highly virulent, fast moving types of cancer that may require resorting to judicious use of chemotherapy and radiation. This is done primarily to slow down the speed of the growth of the malignancy, giving us more time to reinforce the immune system so that it can muster its own resources to combat the cancer. It is unwise to think that chemotherapy and radiation alone will actually cure cancer. The disease is much too complex for that kind of thinking, and it is only the body's own miraculous defense system that can provide a long-term cure. The slower or moderate types of cancer can be handled with surgery, when needed, supported by a whole arsenal of immune-enhancing and cancer-combating substances.

Metabolic Typing determines whether an individual requires a diet lower in protein and fat, and higher in complex carbohydrates (Group I), or a diet higher in protein and fat, and lower in complex carbohydrates (Group II). One of the big breakthroughs that I have discovered in my work through analyzing the files of my clients is that approximately 80% of cancer patients require the lower protein Group I diet, although about 20% of cancer patients need the higher protein Group II diet. Therefore, our nutritional enhancement program for clients with cancer always begins with Metabolic Typing, our most important tool for evaluating blood pH status.

The Importance of a Complementary Approach to Cancer

A deeply troubling article appeared a while ago in the *Townsend Letter for Doctors,* a journal written for, and by, alternative health practitioners. It told the story of a sixty-nine-year-old woman, very committed to holistic medicine, who consulted with four different alternative medical practitioners. She was suffering from a pain in the lower quadrant of her abdomen, and in her legs and hip, which became so severe that she had difficulty moving around, as well as simply enduring it. The four practitioners diagnosed her problem, variously, as a pinched nerve, fibromyalgia, rheumatoid arthritis, or bone atrophy, and each one proceeded to treat her accordingly. Four months went by with no improvement, as her condition worsened. She then sought help from a mainstream doctor who diagnosed her with a very rare type of galloping cancer. By this time, it was too late to save her, and she subsequently died a very painful death.[1]

This person believed strongly in mind, body, and spirit, and a holistic approach to life. While I share her views wholeheartedly, the fact remains that conventional medicine is vitally necessary under certain conditions. Dr. Robert Atkins has earned my admiration for making a distinction between areas where conventional medicine or alternative protocols are better suited.[2] Generally speaking, the holistic approach lends itself best to chronic disease conditions, whereas conventional medicine shines in acute and emergency care, as well as in diagnostic evaluation. One should not merely think in either/or terms, conventional *or* alternative, but rather in terms of complementarity and integration. It is not an either/or choice, but rather a blending of the best each has to offer. Each camp must learn to respect the strengths (and weaknesses) of the other for the benefit of humanity. The needs of the situation must take precedence over attachment to a particular ideology or point of view.

Another case history comes to mind of a patient apparently suffering from TMJ (temporomandibular joint syndrome), a painful condition caused by a defective or partially dislocated temporomandibular joint in the jaw. This individual had been bouncing back and forth from one TMJ specialist to another, but without any real pain relief. I happened to be taking an advanced course on TMJ at the University of California, Berkeley, when the guest lecturer presented this patient to us. He was a young man in his late twenties who was severely depressed. We examined the x-rays and all the investigative work that had already been done by the other TMJ specialists, and we scratched our heads over why no improvement had taken place. The x-rays appeared to be normal. The professor then announced to the class that this had to be more than a TMJ problem, and he sent the patient off to have a complete blood and immune system work-up. The report came back in five days showing extremely high levels of alkaline phosphatase, SGOT, and SGPT, three liver enzymes that, when markedly elevated, indicate a severely compromised immune system. Two weeks later, this young man died of advanced cancer. His problem never had been TMJ, but some of us get so caught up in our specialties that we neglect to see the forest for the trees. Again, we must learn to think in an integrative way.

My Own Bout with Cancer

Another case in point is my own bout with cancer. It all began ten years ago when I was playing tennis, as I have almost every day for the past thirty years. On this particular occasion I was playing doubles, and I lobbed a high return shot to the net person. He slammed the tennis ball back, at an estimated speed of one hundred miles per hour, straight into the inner part of my right thigh. The force of the ball knocked me down, and my leg began to swell severely. One month later, the black-and-blue bruising had gone away, but the swelling remained for many years. As it did not cause me any pain or restrict my movement in any way, I never bothered consulting a doctor. However, when I was seventy-three years old, I glanced down at the swelled mass on my upper thigh and finally decided that it was time to have an MRI. The diagnosis came back as a liposarcoma, a cancerous mutation of the fat cells. At first, I was in complete denial. If it was malignant, why had the tumor not grown and become painful? I was informed that this is the nature of this particular type of cancer, but despite this, it can easily spread (or metastasize) throughout the body. I consented to have surgery, provided I could be awake throughout the procedure, which was performed by two very skillful soft-tumor specialists. It took two and a half hours to remove the growth, and the surgery went remarkably smoothly. Alarmingly, when the biopsy report came back, it was verified to be a stage two sarcoma.

The surgeons wanted me to have bone scans and radiation, and possibly chemotherapy. I declined, and told the doctors I would now handle it my own way. They thought I was crazy, and asked me if I wanted to die. I said no, I wanted to live, but I countered by asking them why I should let them tear down my immune system and undermine my energy with chemotherapy, when its track-record is not very impressive (except for certain cancers, such as leukemia and testicular cancer). They were totally disheartened, but I agreed to return in six months for an evaluation. In the meantime, I initiated my own special cancer protocol, taking over 120 supplements a day, routinely monitoring various metabolic markers. I was very pleased with the results, which showed no indication of metastasis. When I returned for my post-surgical check-up, the doctors scoured the new MRI and blood tests, but were unable to find any evidence of cancer. I am very fortunate and pleased that the tests have remained negative ever since. Hopefully my death, when it comes, will be due to natural causes, not cancer.

I am telling this story because I needed a surgeon to remove the liposarcoma. I had tried many alternatives, but nothing would eliminate the growth. I have already mentioned that I do believe there is a place for chemotherapy and radiation, if only to buy time until non-invasive protocols can be successfully implemented. Buying time for me was not necessary, but the surgery was. My immune system and energy level were excellent at the time of surgery, and continue to be so today. I feel very fortunate that I had been living a healthy lifestyle, eating for my Metabolic Type, exercising, and cultivating a positive mental attitude. My strong immune system kept the cancer from spreading throughout my body; however, it did not prevent me from developing it in the first place. Perhaps genetics played a part, or an improper diet in my earlier days, or having practiced as a dentist—one of the most toxic of professions—for over fifty years.

I am documenting my cancer with the following pathology report:

FIGURE 5-1
Dr. Kristal's
Pathology
Report

THE PERMANENTE MEDICAL GROUP
280 West MacArthur Boulevard, Oakland, CA 94611 Phone: (510)596-6813 FAX: (510) 596-7562

Accession No:	S99-12899	MR Number:	08774811
Accessioned:	08/02/99	Patient:	KRISTAL,HAROLD J
Printed:	08/04/99	DOB/Age/Sex:	06/07/25 (Age: 74) M
Obtained:	08/01/99	Status:	INPATIENT
Service:	ORTHOPEDICS	Coverage code:	SV10N
Facility:	OAKLAND MEDICAL CENTER	Alliance MR #:	
Physician(s):	Richard O'Donnell,MD (SSF ORTH)		

TISSUE SOURCE: RT.THIGH MASS

FINAL DIAGNOSIS:

RIGHT THIGH, EXCISION:
-PLEOMORPHIC LIPOSARCOMA.

/mdj

Gregory J. Rumore, M.D.
(Signed Copy in Chart)
WSP

COMMENT:
This tumor is considered a histologic grade II (of III) or
intermediate grade sarcoma.

PR: TMS.

/mdj

CLINICAL DATA:
7 yr hx R thigh mass. Aspiration c/w hematoma. R/O malignancy.

GROSS DESCRIPTION:
A well-circumscribed, grossly encapsulated, ovoid mass measuring 18 x 10.5 x 7.5 cm.
The outer surface is glistening yellow-tan and smooth. Foci of hemorrhage are
noted. The specimen is oriented by means of three sutures. Prior to sectioning, the
deep margin (single suture) is marked with blue ink, the superficial with yellow ink
and side (triple suture) with black ink. Multiple sections reveal the distal half
of the specimen to consist of homogeneous yellow-tan adipose tissue. The proximal
half is near totally cystic and contains reddish-brown hemorrhagic fluid.
Additional areas of cystic degeneration are noted within the solid area. SLIDE KEY:
(A) Distal end. (B.C.) Deep margin. (D) Hemorrhagic area. (E) Proximal end.
(F.G.) Additional sections, tumor.
GJR/mdj

KRISTAL,HAROLD J   Page 1   Continued on Next Page

Andrew S. Kohler, M.D. Chief	John E. Sawicki, M.D. Assistant Chief
Thomas M. Schmidtknecht, M.D.	Gregory J. Rumore, M.D.
Balaram Puligandla, M.D.	Karen Axelsson, M.D.
Lawrence J. Finkel, M.D.	Geoffrey A. Machin, M.D.

My first reaction when I was told that I had cancer was despair. I was in
shock, and my death seemed imminent. How would I die? Would my death
be painful like that of my father, who succumbed to lung cancer at the age
of forty-three? My emotional state for the next few days was very negative
and despondent. I felt sorry for myself and very angry, even though, in my
heart, I knew that these negative feelings could further damage my health

and my chances for recovery. Then one morning I woke up and said to myself: "Kristal, you have to change the station; you have to change the program. If you are to recover, you need to put into practice the positive orientation that you have been telling your cancer clients about for years."

Within a very short time, my mental attitude changed, and I knew I would survive. This was the start of my new life. My protocol was strict, but I adhered to it with complete discipline. My monitoring tests included the Anti Malignant Antibodies in Serum (AMAS) test, Carcinogenic Embryonic Antigens (CEA), complete liver function panels, comprehensive lipid and immune function assays, natural killer (NK) cell evaluation, and Magnetic Resonance Imaging (MRI). Some of these tests, such as the AMAS, are foreign to the conventional physician, but they helped me monitor improvements in my own condition, as they also do with my clients.

My Own Cancer Supplement Protocol

My own Metabolic Type has always been a Fast Oxidizer (Group II). However, my Sympathetic sub-dominance allowed me to eat large amounts of the fruits and vegetables that are usually restricted on a Group II regimen. During the years preceding my cancer diagnosis, my craving for citrus fruits had magnified, and it was not uncommon for me to eat four organic oranges for a snack. I also craved organic grapefruit juice. My supplement program up to this point had included approximately 40 capsules daily, but after my cancer diagnosis, I began taking 120–140 supplements each day. A large number of these were pancreatic enzymes, averaging 40 per day.

Following is my own supplement program at that time. (Note: proprietary products are shown in italics, followed in parentheses by the name of the company which manufactures them.):

- ∾ *Kristazyme* (PMN; digestive enzymes): 1–2 at the beginning of each meal (3–6 daily);
- ∾ *Formula Three* (PMN; multivitamins/minerals): 12 daily, divided up among my meals;
- ∾ *Essential Balance Oil* (Omega Nutrition): 2 tablespoons daily, with meals;
- ∾ **CoQ10:** 500 milligrams daily, with meals;
- ∾ **Lipoic acid:** 300 milligrams daily, with meals;
- ∾ *Garlic #106* (Kyolic): 12 capsules daily, with meals;

- *Brain Formula* (Body Ammo: 50 mg pregnenolone/50 mg *Ginkgo biloba*/100 mg phosphatidyl serine): 3 capsules with breakfast;
- *MGN-3* (Lane Labs): 6 capsules daily, with meals;
- **Beta 1, 3-Glucan:** 4 capsules daily, between meals;
- *Pancreas Organic Glandular* (Allergy Research Group; pancreatic enzymes): 30–50 daily, taken in six divided doses between meals;
- Vitamin C (mixed mineral ascorbates): 12,000–15,000 mg daily, with meals;
- *AOX/PLX* (Biomed; an antioxidant enzyme mixture containing glutathione peroxidase, superoxide dismutase, catalase, and methionine reductase): 5 daily, later increased to 20 daily, between meals.

Had I known then about the powerful immune system modulators *Moducare* and *ImmPower,* I might also have used one or both of them. In fact, numerous nutritional supplements are available today that have overlapping effects when it comes to enhancing immune function. These range from medicinal mushrooms (such as reishi, shiitake, maitake, and coriolus), to potent antioxidants (such as IP-6, or *AOX/PLX*), to special botanicals or their extracts (such as artemisinin, graviola, or Essiac tea). Each nutritionally oriented practitioner will tend to favor certain compounds that they have found to be efficacious, though practitioners need to stay open to new findings, and be willing to change their recommendations accordingly. The goal, however, is always the same: to empower the immune system to more effectively destroy cancer cells, while simultaneously supporting the health of the rest of the body.

It takes discipline to follow this program, but I was fighting for my life. I knew if I adhered diligently to it, I would beat the cancer. However, almost six weeks after being on the pancreatic enzymes, I started having bouts of nausea. I tried discontinuing the pancreatic enzymes for one day and then resuming them the next, only to find that the nausea would return. This was so devastating to my sense of well-being that I decided to discontinue the pancreatic enzymes entirely, and I instead increased the *AOX/PLX* to 20 daily. I continued this total program for a period of six months until I had complete confirmation that my cancer was in total remission.

I would be remiss if I did not mention that, in addition to nutritional support, there are also several sound alternative medical approaches to cancer treatment. These include insulin potentiation therapy (IPT) and Dr. Stanislaw Burzynski's groundbreaking work with anti-neoplastons (please refer to Resources for contact information). Unfortunately, due to draconian medical regulations that favor only the conventional triad of surgery, radiation, and chemotherapy ("cut, burn, and poison"), physicians risk professional ostracism, serious censure by state medical boards (including the very real threat of the loss of their medical license), and even criminal prosecution for daring to practice these therapies in many states—despite the fact that they have a very impressive track record. It is one thing to protect the public against the charlatans and hucksters who are always around to prey on the vulnerable, but quite another thing to block access to legitimate alternative medical treatments that could save lives. Unfortunately, the medical establishment appears to have a hard time discriminating between the two. The state medical boards, the various national organizations that comprise the cancer establishment, the FDA, and several other state and federal agencies have much to account for in their shameful treatment of courageous physicians who dare to think outside the box, and who put the health of their patients ahead of the medical version of political correctness. (For an in-depth discussion of this dark underbelly to the contemporary cancer scene, I would refer the reader to *The Politics of Cancer Revisited* by Samuel S. Epstein, M.D., and *When Healing Becomes a Crime* by Kenny Ausubel).

The Therapeutic Use of Pancreatic Enzymes

The use of pancreatic enzymes for the treatment of cancer was first suggested in the prestigious medical journal, *The Lancet,* in 1904 by John Beard, a Scottish professor of embryology. Professor Beard advocated the injection of specific amounts of the pancreatic enzymes trypsin and amylopsin into cancer patients. Over the next few years this procedure produced remarkable results, as reported by over forty-three groups of doctors in Europe and the USA. One of these studies was discussed in detail in an article in the *British Medical Journal* in 1907. However, as is so often the case in medical history, the treatment fell from favor after a well-publicized attack by two prominent doctors who claimed it was ineffective, despite the fact that they had only used one-tenth of the dosage recommended by Beard.[3]

However, some sixty years later, William Donald Kelley D.D.S. saw the wisdom in Beard's work. He theorized that cancer was caused, at least in

part, by a deficiency of pancreatic enzymes, a theory suggested by the observation that pancreatic enzyme production declines with age, at the same
time as the incidence of cancer rises. Also, the duodenum—the part of the
small intestine into which the pancreas releases its enzymes—is rarely a
site of cancer formation. Accordingly, Kelley centered his treatment of cancer around the use of pancreatic enzymes, but this time the enzymes were
administered orally and in much higher doses than Beard had originally
stipulated. Kelley, who suffered from pancreatic cancer, was able to cure
himself utilizing these enzymes, and he went on to help thousands of others using this same program. The enzymes were part of a large arsenal of
supplements Kelley recommended, along with appropriate dietary changes
based on his autonomic testing assessment. (Kelley, as you may recall, was
the chief exponent of the Autonomic system, one of the two sub-systems
contained within Metabolic Typing.)

A very plausible explanation for the efficacy of pancreatic enzymes was
provided in 1965 by the research of R. O'Meara of Trinity College in Dublin,
Ireland.[4] O'Meara observed that cancer cells exude clotting factors, which
coat them with fibrin. Fibrin, as its name suggests, is a fibrous protein that
knits together red blood cells to form clots, and is used by the body in the
healing of wounds. However, tumors also use fibrin, in this case to create an
outer layer, or encapsulation, that protects the cancer cells from attack by the
immune system's lymphocytes and cytokines—specifically, cytotoxic T-cells
(CD8), natural killer (NK) cells, and tumor necrosis factor alpha (TNF-alpha).
Pancreatic enzymes are able to break down (or lyse) the fibrin coat, and subsequently, the cancer cells become vulnerable to attack by the immune system's troops of white blood cells. Pancreatic enzymes—with their complement
of trypsin (protease), amylopsin (amylase), and steapsin (lipase)—are generally used to break down food for proper assimilation; but when taken
between meals, they enter the bloodstream and work to "digest" any morbid
matter that is foreign to the body or which compromises its function. (They
are also widely used in mainstream medicine in Germany to counteract arthritis, due to their ability to dissolve calcification in the joints.)

After much deliberation, I have determined that pancreatic enzymes—
which are made from the pancreas of pigs or cows—should be considered a
Group II nutrient. If I am correct in my observation that the majority of
cancer patients are Group I Metabolic Types, then pancreatic enzymes would

be contraindicated for them, especially considering the high dose (between 40 and 80 capsules daily) that is the usual recommendation. It is not unusual for patients to react with intense bouts of nausea from this treatment, which is usually thought to be due to the toxic breakdown of the cancer cells overloading the liver. This may or may not be the reason, but the onslaught of these concentrated Group II nutrients in a body that requires Group I foods will almost certainly contribute to a marked blood pH imbalance. Might not this adverse pH change in the blood be causing the nausea? The therapeutic use of pancreatic enzymes, taken in large numbers at specific intervals several times a day (and, sometimes, night), is a very challenging procedure that requires considerable discipline and motivation. Many of my patients fail to comply because of this difficulty and because of the nausea many of them experience.

Dr. Kelley did, however, have great success in using high doses of pancreatic enzymes as a key component of his extensive supplement regime, and Dr. Nicholas Gonzalez is currently continuing this work with similar positive results in New York City.[5] However, my own program today involves giving only two pancreatic enzymes, along with one plant enzyme *(Kristazyme)*, six times daily on an empty stomach, augmented by a daily dose of 20 caplets of *AOX/PLX*, a unique antioxidant enzyme product. This lower dose of pancreatic enzymes, which is more in accord with Beard's original recommendations, is continued for two to four months, as needed. We discontinue the process when the blood tests come back negative for malignancy, and the client receives a favorable report from their oncologist.

Working with Cancer Patients

Cancer patients come to me at various levels of involvement with conventional treatments, and it is very important for me to know their exact status before I can make any nutritional suggestions and recommendations.

The following evaluations are used:

❧ Metabolic Typing
❧ Diet and Supplement Analysis
❧ Blood Tests
    a) Liver function panel: to determine liver enzyme status;
    b) NK function: to evaluate natural killer (NK) cell competency;

c) AMAS (Anti Malignant Antibodies in Serum): to determine metastasis;

     d) CEA (Carcinogenic Embryonic Antigen): to monitor carcinogensis;

     e) Complete lipid panel: to detect any abnormalities in blood lipids;

- **Weight and Body Fat Percentage**
- **Psychological Evaluation** to determine the client's mental attitude.

The three primary factors needed for defeating malignancy are:

- A proper mental attitude, along with a support network;
- Nutritional support for the immune system;
- Supplements to directly attack the tumor cells.

The Importance of a Positive Mental Attitude

We must not overlook the power of a person's belief system relative to any treatment plan. The mind can act either as a healer or as our own worst enemy. Dr. Carl Simonton, in his inspiring book *Getting Well Again,* cites a case history concerning a new drug, *Krebiozen,* which was touted as the newest cure for cancer. A patient was put on this drug by his doctors, and his recovery was enhanced almost miraculously. This new drug was apparently doing wonders for him, until one day he heard on the radio a report that Krebiozen had been inaccurately assessed as a cure for cancer. After hearing this announcement, his condition rapidly deteriorated, and he finally lost the battle and died.[6] Had he not heard that report, I suspect that his belief in the drug would have given him many more years of life.

Dr. Simonton also cites the case of a wealthy woman who just lost her husband. Her grief was so severe that she too developed cancer, which continued to progress until a new man entered her life. Her happiness with this new relationship actually made her cancer go into remission. However, after a while the money she had inherited from her former husband was used up, and the disappearance of the funds also prompted the disappearance of the man and the subsequent ending of their relationship. She promptly developed cancer again, and soon thereafter lost her battle with the disease.[7] I mention these two cases to demonstrate the power of our belief systems. How many of Dr. Kelley's successful patients held the belief that they could get well with non-invasive techniques? Clearly, the success of any type of medical or nutritional protocol will be greatly amplified by a belief in its efficacy.

The main focus in working with cancer should be on the patient's attitude. People with a "never give up" attitude tend to be survivors. Dr. Carl Simonton's research represents a monumental breakthrough in this area, as does the work of Dr. Bernie Siegel. Might our belief systems contribute more to our recovery than even the best supplement protocol? Dr. Simonton's two case histories certainly suggest this. My advice to all newly diagnosed cancer patients is not to see the diagnosis as a death sentence. Have the will and mental resources to reprogram your mind, and seek the support of loved ones and others who have gone through the process. It will be a journey of growth and healing that will give you a new lease on life. Life is precious. Let us do what we can to fulfill our God-given birthright and our life's destiny.

Non-Hodgkin's Lymphoma

Ricky happened into my office on a referral from one of my clients. He related a very sorry story to me, and I could clearly see that he was quite depressed about his plight. Only in his forties, he had recently developed a pain radiating from his hip to his groin, and a team of doctors diagnosed him with a rare B-cell variety of non-Hodgkin's lymphoma. He was afraid of undergoing the radical treatment that his physicians had laid out for him, partly because he knew the survival rate was quite dismal, so he was interested in looking into alternative treatment options. I emphasized to him that I did not treat cancer or any other disease, but simply provide nutritional support for the body. He appeared very well versed in several alternative cancer treatments, so I told him to get several medical opinions as to the various treatment plans.

On that first visit, when we performed our Metabolic Typing protocol, we discovered he was a Sympathetic type. I outlined a very disciplined dietary and supplement program that he would need to follow. I also explained to him that cancer is not a death sentence; it becomes one only if you let it. I told him how it took me three days after my own cancer diagnosis to get beyond the denial, depression, and anguished questioning as to "why me?". I realized I could never survive with a negative attitude, and so I deliberately worked on changing to a more positive outlook, with the growing confidence that the cancer would not destroy me. If all cancer sufferers could truly cultivate this attitude, survival rates would be greatly enhanced. I truly believe that the mind can be a slayer or a healer. Throughout my first visit with Ricky,

I could see a more confident demeanor take over. When our appointment was over, two and a half hours later, he agreed to obtain a few more opinions, and to bring me a copy of his current laboratory tests. He left with a nutritional plan that would be beneficial both for his Metabolic Type and for shoring up his immune system to help combat the cancer.

I put Ricky on a rigorous regimen of over 100 capsules a day of various supplements during the initial phase, though, at a later visit, I reduced the amount to 60. The initial regimen included eight pancreatic enzymes taken six times daily on an empty stomach (for a total of 48 per day), along with one capsule of the potent digestive enzyme, *Kristazyme.* He also was using the immune enhancers *MGN-3, Moducare,* and Beta 1-3 glucan, along with the powerful antioxidants CoQ10 and lipoic acid, plus extra vitamin C. Together, these nutrients, along with the metabolically balanced diet, helped Ricky's immune system to rally, and to have enough energy to counteract the malignancy.

During the course of that first visit, Ricky had related to me a few business reverses he had experienced (mind as a slayer), but also that he had a lovely one-year-old daughter whom he loved very much, as well as a lovely and supportive wife (mind as a healer). Ricky did his homework and contacted a few cancer specialists. He also sent me copies of all his current blood tests, and he contacted a physician in Mexico familiar with my work in Metabolic Typing. His advice to Ricky was to have six chemotherapy sessions and follow my nutritional protocol with strict discipline. He told him that his oncologist would try to talk him into more than six chemo treatments, but that he should resist, as further treatments would overly weaken his immune system. Ricky decided on this treatment plan, and proceeded with the chemotherapy sessions, along with the diet and supplement regimen, with which he complied 100%. Sure enough, after his sixth chemotherapy, the oncologist ordered him to have more, which Ricky staunchly refused. His energy, sense of well-being, and confidence remained extremely high during this procedure, and although he lost his curly hair, he never got sick.

Upon completion of the course of chemotherapy, Ricky took a series of blood tests, including AMAS, liver function, NK function (a measure of immune competence), and a complete blood panel. I rely heavily on the AMAS test, even though it remains controversial. The AMAS test cannot accurately determine whether or not you have cancer, but it is excellent at detecting metastases. The cancer may still be there, but if the AMAS readings fall into the optimal range, you know your therapy is working. Ricky's AMAS was marginally elevated after the chemo, but a few months later, it came back with optimal readings, and he continued to feel very optimistic (the mind as healer). Finally, his oncologist told him he was in remission, but it was his final AMAS that convinced him that he had won the battle. He hugged me during that visit and told me he was a very lucky man. He reaffirmed his love for his wife and his now two-year-old daughter; I have no doubt that they were both very instrumental in his recovery.

Even though the AMAS was optimal and his oncologists gave Ricky a clean bill of health, cancer cells may still be present in a dormant state in his body. I believe this to be true of my own sarcoma. Both Ricky and I have immune systems strong enough to keep our cancer cells under control. However, we who have survived cancer have to be constantly vigilant about maintaining the highest level of immune competence. Knowing which food and supplements are appropriate for your Metabolic Type is of paramount importance.

Joyce's Story

I would like to tell the story of a very unusual cancer patient. Joyce had been my dental patient for about twenty years before she was diagnosed with incurable, metastasizing colon cancer. In 1992 she told me that her doctors had given her four months to live. They had done everything possible to cure her cancer, including surgery, chemotherapy, and radiation. Joyce had faith in my abilities because five years earlier she had come down with a severe case of bronchitis, and I was able to help her with certain herbs and homeopathic substances. This one successful experience prompted her to seek my advice on her present condition, and she now came to me with the medical prediction of her impending death. She told me that she was not ready to die and was willing to do anything. Back then, my Metabolic Typing protocol was rather primitive in comparison to what it is today, but it was obvious she needed Group I foods and supplements, which she wholeheartedly endorsed. She could not take coffee enemas (a staple of the Kelley anti-cancer protocol) because of her debility, so we gave her a gentle aloe vera/ slippery elm mixture to keep her intestinal tract functional. Basically, all we did for her at that time was to change her diet, give her supplements to help acidify her blood (which was overly alkaline), and antioxidants to prevent a toxin buildup, while maintaining a healthy, operational colon.

She did not die in four months as predicted by her doctors, but lived another eight and a half years until she succumbed, not to cancer but to a heart attack. Joyce never cured her cancer, but she was able to subdue it to the point of peaceful coexistence. From time to time, when one of her tumors enlarged, she would have a little radiation to slow the growth. As new immune-enhancing supplements were developed, we gave them to Joyce. By no means was she cured, but we were able to extend her life and improve its quality. She always looked well and was energetic, and her attitude was always upbeat. She would drive herself to my office and climb up the flight of stairs. If there was one single practical change that helped Joyce the most, I would say it was balancing her blood pH. This enabled her body to more effectively assimilate and utilize her micro- and macronutrients. But her single greatest attribute was her belief that she was not going to let the cancer kill her. We can all learn from Joyce. I certainly have.

Conclusion

An integrated approach combining both conventional and alternative pro-tocols appears to be optimal. In my own case, I needed surgery. Had my cancer been more severe, I would have opted for small amounts of chemotherapy and radiation to buy time until my own immune system could take over. We can only deal with the realities of the here-and-now. Right now, I still have much work to do. My own desire is to help people attain a greater degree of wellness, to be free of pain, and to experience the wonder of living. I hope that these stories will help you understand the importance of a complementary and integrative approach to medicine. It is important for both the conventional doctor and the alternative practi-tioner to acknowledge and respect one other. Conventional doctors have their own expertise concerning the management and treatment of disease, while a metabolically trained practitioner can complement the work of the doctor—who is not extensively trained in nutrition—to help their patients attain optimal health. Success results from an integration of many disci-plines, not a rigid adherence to one.

PROSTATE CANCER: A CRITICAL RE-EVALUATION
~

Once a theory becomes accepted in the medical community, changing it can become a herculean task. Such a situation faces those who ponder the conventional explanation for prostate cancer. Ask almost any medical professional about the cause of prostate cancer, and you will hear that it is due to an excess production of testosterone, which, in turn, changes into its potent and supposedly destructive metabolite dihydrotestosterone (DHT). Based on this belief, one of the primary medical treatment modalities is to short-circuit the production of testosterone and DHT through powerful androgen-suppressing drugs, such as *Casodex* and *Lupron*—a strategy known as an androgen blockade or, less flatteringly, as chemical castration. What is overlooked in this view is an elementary, commonsense question: if prostate cancer is caused by *excess* levels of testosterone, why does it occur primarily in older men, whose testosterone levels are typically reduced, rather than in younger men, whose levels are at their peak? Instead, let us explore an alternative hypothesis: that it may be precisely a *lack* of testosterone, not an excess, that is the primary predisposing factor for prostate cancer, especially in combination with the elevated levels of estrogen that commonly accompany male aging. Our secondary purpose will be to inquire how this understanding affects our approach to the nutritional management and prevention of this disease.

Prostate Cancer: A Brief Overview

Approximately 334,000 new cases of prostate cancer are reported in the U.S. each year. A slow-growing malignancy with a five-year doubling time (the time it takes for the tumor to double in size), prostate cancer often makes an appearance so late in a man's life that treatment becomes moot: the individual would not be expected to live long enough for the cancer to become life-threatening. This often leads more enlightened physicians to take a "watchful waiting" or "hands off" approach to the management of the disease. However, it is increasingly showing up in younger men, sometimes in their early forties; accordingly, prostate cancer is second only to colon cancer as a cause of cancer deaths among U.S. males, claiming 40,000 lives each year.

Like other carcinomas, prostate cancer results from a disordered overgrowth of genetically mutated cells that have lost their differentiated characteristics. Often there are no symptoms in the early stages, though there may be blood in the urine, or even a blockage of the flow of urine from the bladder. It is sometimes detected by a digital rectal exam (DRE), but more commonly by an elevated PSA (prostate specific antigen) test: 0–4 ng/dL is considered normal; over 10 ng/dL is suspect for prostate cancer; and over 20 ng/dL is a definite red flag. If the situation is deemed serious, a biopsy of the tumor may follow. Conventional treatment options include androgen suppressing drugs, radiation, and partial or radical prostatectomy—the surgical removal of the prostate gland that leaves up to 50% of men who undergo the procedure permanently incontinent and/or impotent. Amazingly, even castration is seen as a legitimate medical option.

The Multiple Functions of Testosterone

Testosterone is an anabolic (or tissue building) and androgenic (or masculinizing) hormone that performs a myriad of functions, mediated by cell receptors that are found throughout the entire body. In addition to defining male characteristics in the fetus and the growing male child (the prostate starts out *in utero* as the same cell mass that becomes the uterus in females), testosterone is involved in the production of spermatozoa and the stimulation of libido, as well as the synthesis of protein, which, in turn, makes it a key player in muscle building. Connected to this is its importance in cardiovascular health (as there are more testosterone receptors in the heart than in any other muscle), as well as in bone formation. It also improves oxygen uptake, helps control blood sugar, counteracts adiposity (the deposition of body fat), regulates blood lipids and clotting factors, opposes the stress hormone cortisol, and helps sustain optimal immune function. Furthermore, it also plays a central role in maintaining a man's general energy level, sense of well-being, mood and cognitive abilities, and may well be protective against Alzheimer's disease.[8]

The production of testosterone is initiated when the hypothalamus (the part of the brain that orchestrates endocrine, or hormonal, activity) detects declining levels circulating in the bloodstream. In response it releases gonadotropin-releasing hormone (GnRH) which, in turn, stimulates the pituitary (the hypothalamus' partner in controlling hormone production) to secrete luteinizing hormone (LH), which travels through the bloodstream to the testes, where it stimulates the production of testosterone in the Leydig cells. (A much smaller amount, 5–10% of the total output, is produced in the adrenal glands.) The testosterone is then either used locally to produce spermatozoa in the testes (in the Sertoli cells of the seminiferous tubules)— a process mediated by another pituitary hormone, follicle stimulating hormone (FSH)—or released into the bloodstream to be picked up by receptors elsewhere in the body. Most of the circulating testosterone ends up bound to proteins in the bloodstream (about 75% to sex hormone binding globulin, or SHBG, and 20% or more to albumin and cortisol binding globulin), thereby rendering it largely unavailable to its receptors. The remaining 1–5% that remains biologically active is known as free testosterone.

DHT, the Decline of Testosterone, and the Rise of Estrogen

The free testosterone can itself be transformed into one of three other steroid hormones: the relatively weak androgen, androstenedione; the much stronger testosterone metabolite, dihydrotestosterone (DHT)—stronger because it is able to bind to receptors up to ten times more tightly than testosterone itself; and the potent estrogen, estradiol (E2). Conventional wisdom holds that it is testosterone and DHT (supposedly over-produced by excess testosterone, or by the inability to properly metabolize it) that are largely responsible for stimulating the growth of prostate tumors. Most of the testosterone that enters the prostate gland is indeed converted into DHT (by the enzyme 5-alpha-reductase), where it exerts a powerful anabolic effect on the cells of the prostate, stimulating new growth, and prolonging the life of older cells. As such its effect is rejuvenating.

Can DHT also stimulate the growth of tumors, as is almost universally believed? The supposed overproduction of DHT provides the rationale behind the use of the drug *Proscar* (finasteride), which works by inhibiting the action of 5-alpha-reductase. *Proscar* is used to lessen the symptoms of benign prostatic hypertrophy (BPH), with some limited success (improvement of symptoms for 37% of men after one year), rather than to treat prostate cancer itself. But, if the DHT theory holds water, then *Proscar* should also help prevent the development of prostate cancer. However, a clinical trial, conducted at the University of Southern California with twenty-seven high-risk men taking *Proscar,* showed that eight developed tumors within one year *despite* DHT levels that had been significantly lowered below baseline. By comparison, only one man in the twenty-five-person control group developed a tumor.[9] The implication is that *Proscar* (or, by extension, reduced levels of DHT) may actually *increase,* rather than decrease, the risk of developing prostate cancer.

An alternate view holds that DHT only becomes a problem when it combines with excess levels of estrogen, possibly because—unlike testosterone itself—DHT does not help control estrogen levels.[10] As men age, not only do their testosterone levels tend to drop, but also their estrogen levels tend to rise. Just as optimal progesterone levels oppose estrogen in a woman's body, thereby offsetting the destructive phenomenon of estrogen dominance, so too does testosterone control estrogen in a man's body. When testosterone levels start to decline, there is often a parallel rise in estrogen. It is a remarkable, if little known, fact that men in their mid fifties generally produce more estrogen than women in the same age group![11] The decline of testosterone (from a high of 800–1200 ng/dL in the late teens to as low as 200 ng/dL later in life) takes the form of either primary or secondary hypogonadism (or under-production by the testes). Primary hypogonadism is due to declining capacity in the Leydig cells in the testes, and is clinically indicated by unusually high blood levels of circulating gonadotrophins (the hormones LH and FSH that stimulate the function of the testes), as the pituitary tries in vain to jump-start the failing Leydig cells by pumping out more of these hormones. Secondary hypogonadism, which may be the more common of the two scenarios, involves subnormal release of LH and FSH by a sluggish pituitary gland. Primary hypogonadism can be treated medically by the administration of testosterone, and secondary hypogonadism by another hormone called chorionic gonadotrophin (CG) which functions similarly to LH in stimulating the Leydig cells.[12]

While either form of hypogonadism is sufficient to initiate the symptoms of andropause, or "male menopause" (most notably, failing energy and libido), rising estrogen levels can further complicate the picture. A certain percentage of testosterone is converted into estrogen throughout a man's life by the enzyme aromatase (a process known as aromatization), possibly to prevent an over-production of testosterone. As men enter their middle years, production of aromatase rises, and along with it estrogen levels. This tends to increase adiposity (especially of the apple-shaped/love-handles/spare-tire/pot-belly variety), but fat cells themselves further concentrate aromatase, initiating a vicious cycle of ever increasing estrogen production. Estrogen displaces testosterone on its receptor sites and—because the two hormones are very closely related in chemical structure—it tricks the hypothalamus into thinking that testosterone levels are sufficiently high, thereby reducing (or down-regulating) further testosterone production. Whereas the ratio between testosterone and estrogen might have previously been around 50:1, now it might drop to less that 10:1. Ironically, higher estrogen levels also stimulate the production of more SHBG (sex hormone binding globulin), which aggressively binds up the diminishing amount of circulating free testosterone. This situation is even further exacerbated by alcohol consumption, which itself increases estrogen production (contributing to the infamous "beer belly"), as well as by the almost ubiquitous presence of xenoestrogens (quasi-estrogenic compounds) in the environment, found in such substances as pesticides, industrial pollutants, and plastics. The xenoestrogens, which have been steadily building up in the environment over the last fifty years and which now number over 70,000 different chemicals, may well be responsible for the increasing appearance of prostate cancer in younger men—a phenomenon almost completely unknown until the later decades of the twentieth century.[13]

Unopposed estrogen is well-known for its tumor promoting action. The question remains: does DHT play any active role at all in this process? A French endocrinologist, Bruno de Lignieres, claims that DHT may actually have a *protective,* even therapeutic role, precisely because—unlike testosterone—it cannot be aromatized into estrogen.[14] This is supported by laboratory trials in which rats given DHT demonstrated a remarkable 50% reduction in the development of prostate tumors. Furthermore, patients with prostate cancer typically have lower levels of DHT than cancer-free individuals.[15] Add to this the lifetime work of the legendary, if controversial, Danish physician Jens Møller who, until his death in 1989, successfully treated thousands of men with high doses of testosterone for various advanced cardiovascular conditions (usually related to diabetes) without *ever* seeing prostate cancer develop in *any* of his patients.[16] Taken together, this evidence strongly suggests that it is unopposed estrogen, rather than excess testosterone or even DHT, that appears to be the culprit in promoting the unrestrained growth of prostate cells that leads to cancer. This might also explain why the 5-alpha-reductase inhibitors, like *Proscar,* may actually *increase* the risk for developing prostate cancer: by blocking the conversion of testosterone to DHT (which cannot be converted into estrogen), these drugs may indirectly encourage it to be converted into yet more estrogen.

Hormones for the Prevention and Treatment of Prostate Cancer

What seems clear from all of this is that testosterone needs to be maintained at optimal levels, and estrogen held in check, to prevent the development of prostate cancer. Functional laboratory assessments—either blood, urine, or saliva tests—should be used in middle-aged and older men to monitor levels of these key hormones. (Saliva tests are generally thought to be more reliable than blood tests because they measure only free levels of hormones, which are not accurately detectable in serum. Hormones are fat-soluble and therefore travel through the bloodstream attached to the fatty membranes of the red blood cells, rather than in the water-soluble medium of the serum, which is what is assayed in blood tests). If necessary, supplementation with natural testosterone should be considered. As testosterone is a controlled substance, its use does not fall under the mandate of a nutritionist, and it would need to be prescribed by a physician. It should preferably be used transdermally (in a cream base that is absorbed through the skin), and in its natural form (i.e. perfectly matching the molecular structure of human testosterone) rather than in its synthetic forms (such as methyltestosterone or testosterone enanthate). Synthetic hormones carry a risk of side effects—which can be potentially serious—that is rarely found to any significant degree with natural hormones.

Another option would be the use of androstenedione. This mildly androgenic testosterone precursor (which is available without a prescription) has received some bad press, partly because its use by baseball superstar Mark McGuire raised legitimate concerns that teenage boys and young men would be tempted to emulate his lead, thereby raising their already naturally high testosterone levels to potentially dangerous levels (as *any* hormone elevated significantly beyond its normal reference range is potentially dangerous); and partly because the liver readily converts it into one of the potent forms of estrogen, estrone (E1). However, in its transdermal form it bypasses the liver and is slowly released into the bloodstream—as distinct from the unnaturally rapid boost that follows oral ingestion. Some companies marketing transdermal androstenedione creams compound it with progesterone to minimize its conversion into estrone. Even more desirable might be androstenediol, a closely related testosterone precursor that cannot be aromatized into estrogen. (See Resources for availability of these compounds.) It is wise to periodically re-test hormone levels once every few months when using these or other hormone replacement products.

Transdermal progesterone cream is also currently being explored, both as a preventative measure and therapeutically for men with active prostate cancer (in doses of 4–12 mg/day, as determined by saliva assays). *In vitro* (test tube) studies have shown that while estrogen stimulates the activity of the tumor-promoting oncogene BCL2 in prostate cells (as well as in breast and uterine cells), progesterone (and also testosterone) inhibit its activity by activating the P53 protector gene. (Interestingly, insulin also stimulates the growth of cancer cells, adding yet another reason for eating a glycemically controlled diet). While it is too early to be definitive about its long-term value, preliminary anecdotal reports from an on-going human clinical trial using transdermal progesterone, conducted through the University of California at Santa Barbara, are encouraging.[17] Progesterone can be safely used to oppose the destructive effects of elevated estrogen, though questions still remain about the use of other hormones for the same purpose. While testosterone and its precursors (androstendione, androstenediol, DHEA) are protective against the initiation of prostate cancer, it remains a theoretical possibility that giving them to men with active prostate cancer *may* encourage more rapid growth of cancer cells, though no hard data exists to support this theory. The same concern has been expressed about human growth hormone (hGH)—which, like testosterone ad the other androgens, is a powerful anabolic (or growth promoting) agent—and also about thyroid hormone, though controversy continues to rage on these issues.[18] Until more is definitively known, erring on the side of caution seems wise.

Nutritional Options

Many nutrients are known to benefit the health of the prostate: the mineral zinc and the omega-3 essential fatty acids (as found in flax seeds and oily fish) seem to be particularly important, as well as the carotenoid lycopene (found primarily in cooked tomatoes), the trace mineral selenium, the pro-hormone vitamin D, and the plant lipid beta-sitosterol. The well-known herb saw palmetto (itself a significant source of beta-sitosterol) is known to relieve the symptoms of BPH (benign prostatic hypertrophy) by inhibiting the action of 5-alpha-reductase, but unlike *Proscar,* it appears to gently modulate rather than blindly suppress its action. What implications, if any, this has for prostate cancer are not clear. High doses of CoQ10 (400–600 mg/day), which have demonstrated a pronounced benefit in several breast cancer cases, may also be of use.[19]

Soy isoflavones (primarily genistein and daidzein) and the proprietary herbal product *PC-SPES* have both been very popular among alternatively minded prostate cancer patients. Both exhibit estrogen-mimicking proper-ties and, while this may seem as if it would exacerbate estrogen levels, the milder phytoestrogens present in these products seem to work by displac-ing the stronger endogenous (self-produced) estrogens on the receptor sites. However, controversy continues to surround the use of powerful phytoe-strogens (plant estrogen mimics), and their use should be considered exper-imental and approached with caution. (*PC-SPES* was recently removed from the market when it was found to contain pharmaceutical hormones and other contaminants.) There are numerous anecdotal reports that suggest that, if used at therapeutic doses for extended periods, they may lead to tem-porary impotence, which is resolved when their use is discontinued. Also, therapeutic doses of phytoestrogens are contraindicated for breast cancer survivors, as they may actually encourage the re-growth of tumor cells; thus, given that prostate cancer, like breast cancer, appears to be estrogen-driven, the use of phytoestrogens may, over time, prove to be counterproductive.

Indole compounds, distributed widely in vegetables of the brassica or cruciferous family (broccoli, cauliflower, Brussels sprouts, cabbage, kale, bok choy, turnip, etc.), show tremendous promise in the prevention and treat-ment of estrogen-driven cancers. Researcher Maria Bell, M.D. recently announced the astonishing results of a randomized, placebo-controlled, dou-ble-blind trial (the gold standard of clinical trials) showing a 40–50% remis-sion in patients in stages 2 and 3 of a particular form of cervical cancer known as cervical intraepithelial neoplasia (CIN). This remarkable turnaround occurred after only twelve weeks of supplementing with the indole extract indole-3-carbinol (I3C). How these data can be extrapolated to prostate cancer remains unknown, but it is of interest to note that the proposed method of action was to divert estrone (E1) into its benign metabolite 2-hydroxyestrone, rather than into the tumor promoting 16-alpha-hydroxyestrone form. Dr. Jonathan Wright, one of the most respected holistic physicians in the US, postulates that an imbalance of the ratio between these two estrone metabolites may also play a role in the development of prostate cancer; happily their ratios can be easily and accurately tested by a simple urine test.[20] The active indoles found in the brassica family are indole-3-carbinol (I3C), diindolylmethane (DIM) (composed of a coupled pair of I3C molecules), and ascorbigen (I3C bonded to ascorbic acid, or vitamin C). While any of these substances may be used alone supplementally, they appear to work synergistically in combination. Science is once again validating what your grandmother always told you: eat your vegetables!

Numerous botanicals and other natural substances are also thought to raise testosterone levels. Though clinical experience would seem to bear this out, most have not yet been subjected to rigorous scientific scrutiny. These include: deer antler velvet (derived from the soft outer portion of antlers that are sloughed off annually by male deer); muira puama *(Ptychopetalum olacoides)*, a Brazilian herb popularly known as Potency Wood; horny goat weed *(Epimedium sagittatum);* tribulus *(Tribulus terrestris);* panax ginseng; and the Peruvian herb maca *(Lepidum meyenii)*, which appears to be equally beneficial as an endocrine tonic for both men and women (probably by acting on the hypothalamus). Many, if not all, of these substances work as endocrine modulators, rather than as direct testosterone stimulants, which may represent a superior long-term strategy, as they encourage the body to "find its own level" rather than superimposing a predetermined dosage from the outside.

Other substances that may be of benefit to prevent or counteract prostate cancer include:

❧ **Artemisinin:** an extract of the herb artemesia *(Artemesia annua)* that combines with the iron found in tumor cells to produce a peroxide reaction that kills malignant cells, without harming healthy ones;[21]

❧ **Crinum:** a species of Vietnamese waterlily, crinum *(Crinum latiforlium)* enhances the ability of the immune system to counteract prostate enlargement and tumor growth;[22]

❧ **Chrysin:** a bioflavonoid extracted from passionflowers, which inhibits the action of aromatase, thereby interrupting the transformation of testosterone (as well as DHEA and, presumably, androstenedione) into estrogen;

❧ **Graviola:** *(Annona muricata)*, an Amazonian rainforest herb which has been shown in laboratory studies, conducted under the auspices of the National Cancer Institute, to be cytotoxic to various cancer cell types, including prostate adenocarcinoma; unlike chemotherapy drugs, which it appears to match or even exceed in potency, graviola only targets malignant cells without harming healthy ones;[23] however, there are anecdotal reports of graviola elevating PSA levels, raising the possibility that elevated PSA levels are a sign of the immune system rallying against the malignancy, rather than a direct sign of the malignancy itself;[24]

❧ *Poly MVA:* a liquid compound containing the metallic mineral element palladium, complexed with the antioxidant lipoic acid and various other nutrients, which appears to selectively target and destroy malignant cells by denaturing their proteins.[25]

Conclusion

Though much remains to be discovered about the role of hormones in the initiation (or pathogenesis) of prostate cancer, it is becoming increasingly clear that lowered testosterone and elevated estrogen levels—and the corresponding disruption of the ratio between the two—appears to play an important, if not central role. As such it would be prudent for middle-aged and older men to take steps to either prevent or reverse this scenario.

CHAPTER 6

A Potpourri of Nutritional Information

THE REVERSE EFFECT

Almost every day I receive advertisements for new products touted as panaceas for all our ills and ailments. These vitamins, minerals, herbs, and specialty products are said to boost energy, melt fat, eliminate pain, and cure everything from arthritis to impotence. The colorful flyers often include ecstatic testimonials from people whose migraines, depression, obesity, pain, wrinkles, and even cancer have disappeared overnight, thanks to the new miracle product. These people declare that they are now in vibrant good health and are enjoying life more than ever before. We all want to feel this way, so no wonder these advertisements are so effective at persuading people to buy what are sometimes high-priced and frivolous products. Of course, some of them do have very real merit for specific conditions. By and large, however, they do not measure up to the extravagant claims made for them. We must not be taken in by advertisers whose primary mission is, after all, to sell their product.

In my own practice, patients constantly bring me articles and flyers about marvelous new products they are eager to try. I usually advise caution. Even if a given product is beneficial to your friend, it may be harmful to you. The crucial first step is to determine your Metabolic Type in order to know how each substance will affect your chemical balance or imbalance. Any given food or supplement could move your system toward greater equilibrium and health, or toward greater imbalance and disease. It is impossible to predict which will happen without knowing your Metabolic Type.

One of my goals as a nutritionist is to recommend as few supplements as possible. What that means in practice will vary from individual to individual, and I do not shy away from recommending as many supplements as I see fit. However, I firmly believe that food is always your best medicine, and no amount of supplements—even good ones—can compensate for a bad diet. When the body is properly nourished and in balance, the blood will be at its ideal pH level, and then all metabolic systems will operate with ease and efficiency. However, foods and supplements that are inappropriate for your Metabolic Type can move the blood away from its ideal pH so that it becomes too acid or too alkaline. The further it gets away from the ideal pH, the more discomfort, dysfunction, and disease will result.

We have explored in detail the idea that two of the four Metabolic Types (Fast Oxidizers and Sympathetics) have a tendency to be too acid, and two have a tendency to be too alkaline (Slow Oxidizers and Parasympathetics). Each needs to be helped toward the ideal pH that lies between these two extremes. In order to do this, it is crucial to understand the dynamics of how various foods and supplements act upon each type of metabolism. Each food or supplement ingested will tend to make the blood more acid *or* more alkaline, in varying degrees. Furthermore, as we have seen repeatedly, the same food will have opposite effects in members of the two dominance systems, the Oxidative and the Autonomic: foods that acidify the Oxidative types (Fast and Slow Oxidizers) will alkalize the Autonomic types (Sympathetics and Parasympathetics), and vice versa. Some will change the blood pH substantially, while others will have more moderate effects.

When we test an individual to determine their Metabolic Type, we are able to recommend the ideal diet and supplement protocol for that type. This is not a rigid regime, but it does include a list of foods among which a person can choose. We also recommend supplements appropriate to the person's Metabolic Type, as well as to their specific health condition. Recommending the same supplement for everyone is misguided in my opinion, and a misuse of the product. What is helpful for one person can easily have a reverse effect on another, and may actually do harm by creating or exacerbating an acid or alkaline imbalance. When the blood pH is driven away from its optimal value, any number of ills can result, ranging from subtle and minor to major and debilitating. To reiterate one of the main themes of this book, no diet or supplement program is ideal for everyone.

Nutrition is nutrition is nutrition. But one person's healthy food can be another person's poison. This is why it is so important to ascertain each person's Metabolic Type before designing a nutritional program. Without this knowledge we are likely to suggest nutrients and supplements which can be useless or, worse, potentially harmful. Knowledge about nutrition doubles every few years, and thus to maintain one's expertise in the subject is an ongoing challenge. For example, a book called *The Reverse Effect*, written in the 1980s by Walter A. Heiby, tells how vitamins and minerals can promote health or cause disease. We all know that vitamins and minerals can promote health, but can they also cause disease? It is Heiby's thesis that they can, a phenomenon he calls the Reverse Effect.[1] To support his thesis he cites 4,821 references.

As I read the book, which is an excellent overall work on nutrition, I realized that the author was apparently not aware of the research on metabolic individuality that explains why a given nutritional substance may help one individual, have no effect on a second person, and have a negative impact on a third. How can this be? The answer lies in metabolic individuality. Just as one person's food is another person's poison, the same supplements can affect different people in different ways. We now know that nutrients change the acid/alkaline balance of our blood, but in variable ways. For example, calcium will have an alkaline effect on the Oxidative types but an acid effect on the Autonomic types. This same variable effect applies to magnesium, potassium, vitamins A, B, C, D, and E, and most of the supplements known today. Walter Heiby saw this happening over and over again, but he did not understand why. Metabolic Typing, however, offers an explanation. Had Heiby known that the ideal blood pH was 7.46, he might have realized that any supplement that causes the blood pH to deviate too far above (alkaline) or below (acid) the optimal level will impair the individual's ability to assimilate and properly utilize macro- and micronutrients. When this happens, pH imbalances set the stage for disease symptoms to appear.

We have already discussed the example of calcium, which is commonly recommended for osteoporosis. While it may be helpful to one person, it can actually increase bone loss in another. The reason for this is that calcium acidifies the blood of certain individuals (Sympathetics and Parasympathetics) but alkalizes the blood of others (Fast and Slow Oxidizers). For example, if Slow Oxidizers, who are already overly alkaline, take calcium, they will be made even more alkaline. To try to redress this imbalance, the body pulls other minerals out of the bones—which serve as a storehouse of minerals— to buffer this overly alkaline condition in the bloodstream. Unfortunately, this leads to a further undermining of the integrity of the bones. Therefore, it is important to know your Metabolic Type to understand whether calcium will be helpful (as it will be for Fast Oxidizers and Parasympathetics) or detrimental (as it can be for Slow Oxidizers or Sympathetics).

What had confounded Walter Heiby in his book *The Reverse Effect*, despite all of his admirable research, is clearly understandable from the viewpoint of Metabolic Typing. Thus we can see how vital it is to know our own Metabolic Type so that we can tailor our diet and supplement program to what is most appropriate for the way our own body actually works, instead of being at the mercy of whatever dietary philosophy happens to be in vogue.

THE AMINO ACID CONNECTION

Amino acids are the building blocks of protein. They are strung together, in various configurations, into short chains known as peptides or longer chains known as polypeptides ("many peptides"). The way the amino acids are sequenced in these chains determines the shape and properties of the proteins. Proteins are generally broken down into their constituent amino acids during the digestive process, though it has been discovered in recent years that some small-chain peptides are absorbed intact into the bloodstream. Amino acids are in constant demand for a host of bodily functions, including: the growth and repair of tissues, such as muscle, skin, bone, hair, connective tissue, and internal organs; the formation of red and white blood cells; the synthesis of enzymes, hormones, and brain chemicals (neurotransmitters); the transportation of other nutrients in the bloodstream; and as an energy source.

Amino acids are divided into two main classification groups: *essential* and *non-essential*. These terms do not refer to their relative importance, as common sense might suggest, but to whether or not the body is able to synthesize them internally. The eight essential amino acids are those which must be consumed daily in the diet (or through supplementation) to supply the body's needs. Non-essential amino acids are those which the body is able to

Essential Amino Acids

Isoleucine, leucine, lysine, methionine, phenylalanine, threonine, tryptophan, valine

Non-essential Amino Acids

Alanine, arginine, asparagine, aspartic acid, cysteine, cystine, GABA (gamma-aminobutyric acid), glutamic acid, glutamine, glycine, histidine, hydroxyproline, proline, serine, taurine, tyrosine

Three other sub-groups can also be identified:

Conditionally Essential Amino Acids

These are defined as amino acids that are generally non-essential but which become essential under specific conditions, such as during infancy (arginine, taurine, histidine), during certain illnesses, or under conditions of prolonged stress.

Intermediate Amino Acids

Amino acids that are synthesized temporarily during the metabolic processing of other amino acids; examples include homocysteine, citrulline, and ornithine.

Secondary Amino Acids

Various other amino acids that are present in the body in small amounts; very little is known about what functions they perform, if any.

synthesize from essential amino acids and other nutrients. Foods that contain all eight of the essential amino acids—such as meat, fish, eggs, and dairy products—are referred to as complete proteins; foods that lack one or more essential amino acid are called incomplete proteins. Almost all plant foods are incomplete proteins; for example, legumes are typically low in lysine, and grains are typically low in methionine. Vegetarians need to be especially vigilant to ensure that they consume all eight essential amino acids on a daily basis, or else serious health consequences may follow.

The body itself also synthesizes special combinations of amino acids, or peptides, which are formed by the bonding of two or more amino acids. The best known of these is glutathione—a tri-peptide consisting of cysteine, glycine, and glutamic acid—which is the body's most powerful internal antioxidant, playing a crucial role in the ability of the cells and the liver to detoxify potentially harmful substances.

Carnitine, which is formed from lysine and methionine in the presence of nutrient co-factors, is often listed as a non-essential amino acid, but it lacks the amino group, one of the two groups of molecules that chemically defines an amino acid. This has led to some disagreement among experts as to whether or not it technically qualifies as an amino acid, and, in some ways, it more closely resembles the B-vitamin choline than an amino acid.[2] However we choose to classify it, carnitine is an exceptional nutrient with many properties, including promoting weight loss, enhancing energy production and athletic endurance, and improving circulation and general cardiovascular functioning.

Note that amino acids are generally used supplementally in their L- (*levo* or left) forms, rather than in their D- (*dextro* or right) forms. (The L- and the D- refer to different asymmetrical forms of the same molecule, which impart different properties.) Occasionally, the hybrid DL- form is used, the most common of which is the analgesic DL-phenylalanine. The L- form of amino acids are properly written with L- preceding the name of the amino acid (e.g. L-arginine) but, for the sake of simplicity and to avoid repetition, we refer to them here without the L- (e.g. arginine). Whereas protein foods (such as meat, fish, eggs, and dairy products) require special digestive enzymes (called proteases) to break the protein down into its constituent amino acids, free-form (or isolated) amino acids are absorbed without the need for enzymes, and are generally some of the easiest of supplements for the body to assimilate. However, co-factors, such as vitamins and minerals, are needed within the body to help the amino acids perform their proper functions.

Following are some of the numerous uses, both metabolic and therapeutic, for the various amino acids:

∾ **Arginine:** helps maintain weight and stimulates muscle growth; enhances libido; increases sperm count and motility; assists wound healing; acts as a precursor to nitric oxide and human growth hormone (hGH); may enhance lymphocyte (immune) activity; may help to inhibit tumor formation.

∾ **Aspartic acid** and **Asparagine:** provide brain stimulation.

∾ **Cysteine:** critical to proper liver functioning; detoxifies carcinogens, heavy metals, and other dangerous chemicals; antioxidant; primary component of glutathione; promotes healthy skin.

∾ **GABA:** calming; anti-anxiety; anti-epileptic.

∾ **Glutamic acid:** precursor to glutamine and GABA; raises blood sugar levels in people with hypoglycemia.

∾ **Glutamine:** suppresses sugar and carbohydrate cravings; counteracts hypoglycemia; nourishes and heals the lining of the gastrointesinal tract; counteracts diarrhea.

∾ **Glycine:** reduces sugar cravings; promotes wound healing; is calming in manic depression and epilepsy.

∾ **Histidine:** reduces high blood pressure; relieves allergic reactions; facilitates orgasm; helps in the management of rheumatoid arthritis.

∾ **Hydroxyproline** and **Proline:** key components of collagen, the fibrous protein that forms the body's connective tissue.

∾ **Leucine, Isoleucine, and Valine** (collective known as branched chain amino acids, or BCAAs): promote muscle growth and repair.

∾ **Lysine:** controls herpes simplex; acts as a carrier for calcium transport; a key precursor of carnitine.

∾ **Methionine:** anti-depressant; precursor to cysteine, taurine, and SAMe (S-adenosyl-methionine); counteracts allergies; protects against radiation.

∾ **Phenylalanine:** stimulates the brain; is a precursor of tyrosine and adrenaline; relieves chronic pain.

∾ **Taurine:** is calming; lowers blood pressure; supports the pumping action of the heart; protects the retina and neurons; antioxidant; assists in detoxification; anti-convulsant.

∾ **Threonine:** stimulates immune function.

∾ **Tryptophan:** combats depression, insomnia and various mental disorders; produces serotonin and melatonin.

∾ **Tyrosine:** is a precursor of thyroxine (thyroid hormone) and several stimulating (or excitatory) neurotransmitters (including dopamine); enhances energy production; anti-depressant.

Amino acids are taken therapeutically in amounts ranging from 500 mg to several grams per day, depending on the purpose for which they are being used. They are usually taken on an empty stomach, at least thirty minutes before a meal, to prevent other amino acids found in food from competing with them for absorption. It is generally recommended that an individual work with a nutritionist or holistically oriented physician when taking amino acid supplements. (For more information on these and other therapeutic uses for amino acids, refer to *The Amino Revolution* by Robert Erdmann, or *The Healing Nutrients Within* by Eric Braverman.)

THE IMPORTANCE OF FATTY ACIDS
~

One of the questions most frequently asked in our clinic is: "Why do I need to take the Omega Nutrition *Essential Balance Oil* that you recommend?" Unlike most other supplements, this oil—or a comparable product—is recommended to *all* Metabolic Types, albeit in differing amounts. So why, indeed, do we universally recommend it?

Oils are liquid forms of fat and, as such, they are subjected to the unfortunate stigma our society visits upon this most misunderstood of nutrients. Fats (or, more technically, lipids) have been vilified largely because of the association the word has with body fat (adipose tissue), America's public enemy number one. Yet without fat in our diet and in our bodies, life would literally be unsustainable. Fats make up the membranes of every single cell in our bodies, including the cells in the eyes that are right now reading these words, and the brain that is comprehending them. In fact, approximately 60% of the brain is comprised of fat. One much misunderstood lipid—cholesterol— provides the raw material for *all* our adrenal hormones, including the sex hormones estrogen, progesterone, and testosterone, while other lipids play vital roles in energy production and storage, brain and heart function, nervous system activity, transport of fat-soluble vitamins, enzyme regulation, control of inflammation, and cell membrane integrity. Fats also provide us with the feeling of satiety after eating a meal, and, contrary to popular misconception, normal consumption of healthy fats does not make us fat—although an excess can do so, especially for the Group I Metabolic Types (Slow Oxidizers and Sympathetics). It is sugar and starchy carbohydrates, not fats, that are chiefly responsible for expanding waistlines.

The main types of dietary fat are saturated, monounsaturated, and polyunsaturated—biochemical terms that refer to the amount of hydrogen atoms that are filling or "saturating" their carbon chains. Saturated fats contain the most hydrogen atoms, making them more stable than the unsaturated fats and, therefore, less vulnerable to the dangerous process of oxidation. Fats can either be referred to by their full name (e.g. saturated fat) or by adding the suffix -*ate* onto the end of their name (e.g. saturate). Most foods contain a mixture of these fatty acids—fatty acids are the building blocks of fats, just as amino acids are the building blocks of protein— but are generally classified by the dominant one. Butter, for example, is commonly classified as a saturated fat, even though it contains nearly 30% oleic acid, the very same monounsaturated fatty acid that is so revered in olive oil.[3]

Saturated Fats

An excess of saturated fat (which is found primarily in animal foods) has been circumstantially—but by no means conclusively—associated with atherosclerosis (hardening of the arteries) and heart disease, and our whole culture has been inculcated with the erroneous belief that saturated fat only contributes to ill-health and has no beneficial properties—even though serious lipid and cardiovascular researchers are far from unanimous in this opinion.[4] Saturated fats actually have many beneficial functions in the body, including the crucial roles of giving strength to the cell membranes (a function they share with cholesterol), and lubricating the lungs.[5] If not enough saturated fats are consumed in the diet, the body will actually synthesize them to assure that there are enough to meet all of its metabolic needs. Similarly, the body can use saturates as the raw material to synthesize oleic acid, the "heart healthy" monounsaturated omega-9 fatty acid.[6] Saturates also facilitate the enzymatic conversion of the omega-3 alpha-linolenic acid into its active long-chain forms, EPA (eicosapentaenoic acid) and DHA (docosahexaenoic acid),[7] a process hindered by the excess consumption of the omega-6 linoleic acid, which is concentrated in the commonly used vegetable oils, such as corn, safflower, sunflower, and soy oils.[8]

Saturates are particularly important for the Group II Metabolic Types (Fast Oxidizers and Parasympathetics) who require a higher intake of all fats than the Group I Metabolic Types (Slow Oxidizers and Sympathetics). So long as they are not eaten to excess, and are balanced by the essential fatty acids (especially the omega-3 fats), saturated fats are a healthy food, despite all the propaganda to the contrary. Interestingly, the original studies that claimed to prove the dangers of saturated fats were not performed with naturally saturated fats, but with artificially saturated vegetable oils, produced through the dangerous process of partial hydrogenation.[9] Other studies were performed on vegetarian animals like rabbits that are unable to metabolize saturated fats.[10] As we shall see, partially hydrogenated fats (which contain highly toxic *trans* fatty acids) behave very differently in the body than naturally saturated fats (which do *not* contain *trans* fats, except for tiny amounts in a different, safe, form in some dairy products).

There are several different saturated fatty acids, the most common of which are the long-chain stearic, palmitic, and myristic acids. Two kinds of saturates with special properties are: medium chain triglycerides (MCTs), which are sold in supplement form to athletes to increase short-term energy production and which are not stored as body fat; and lauric acid, which has powerful antimicrobial and immune-enhancing properties—accounting, no doubt, for its significant presence in human breast milk. Both of these fatty acids are found in coconut oil (a whopping 49% of which is lauric acid); if it is not refined (and unfortunately it often is), coconut oil—also known as coconut butter, due to its semi-solid consistency at room temperature—is a very useful cooking oil. Saturates are the *only* oils that are stable under normal heat conditions, which is why—in the form of lard, coconut, or palm oil—they were almost universally used as cooking fats in traditional cultures. Butter is fairly stable under heat, because it is 50% saturated. The monounsaturates (primarily olive oil) are the next most stable oils when heated, but significantly less than the saturates, and should never be more than lightly heated. The polyunsaturates, which are commonly used as cooking oils (corn, safflower, sunflower, and soy oils) are rapidly oxidized by heat, and should never be used in stove-top cooking. The one exception is sesame oil, a hybrid polyunsaturated/monounsaturated oil (43% and 41%, respectively), which contains a potent antioxidant (sesamin) that helps to protect the fatty acids from forming toxic lipid peroxides when exposed to heat. A good quality coconut oil (such as Omega Nutrition's *Coconut Oil*) is by far the best choice for a cooking oil, followed by butter, olive and sesame oils. Canola oil is not recommended, even though it is predominantly monounsaturated, primarily because the rapeseed crop from which it is produced has been genetically engineered, and/or the oil has been heavily refined. Also, its modest omega-3 content (10% or less) renders it unsuitable for cooking. (Please see the section on Oils in Chapter 3.)

Monounsaturated Fat

Monounsaturated ("mono-unsaturated") fat has been highly touted for its well-established ability to lower serum cholesterol and to support the health of the heart, while helping to balance blood sugar levels and regulate insulin metabolism.[11] Its best known form is oleic acid (or omega-9), the predominant fatty acid found in olive oil, avocados, and most nuts (with macadamia nuts an especially good source). Excellent though this oil is, it is not considered *essential*—a technical term that, as we saw with amino acids, refers to a substance that the body cannot synthesize from other ingredients, and must therefore obtain through the diet. Monounsaturates, such as olive oil, are relatively stable under moderate heat, but great care should be taken not to burn them. Not only is the burned oil dangerous in itself, as burning creates highly toxic lipid peroxides and *trans* fats in the oil, but so too is the smoke that it gives off, which is potentially carcinogenic.[12] If you do accidentally burn an oil, open a window and leave the room immediately; then, after the fumes have cleared, discard the burned oil. Monounsaturates are best used cold or lightly heated.

Polyunsaturates

Only two fatty acids are considered essential (as defined above), and both are polyunsaturates ("poly-unsaturates"). These are omega-6 (linoleic acid), which is found widely in nuts, seeds, whole grains, and vegetables; and omega-3 (alpha-linolenic acid), which is found primarily in flax seeds and in cold-water fish, as well as, to a lesser degree, in walnuts and green leafy vegetables. Both are also found in animal products, but are much more concentrated in wild game and free-range animals (that are pastured on grass) than in factory-farmed, feed-lot animals. Where saturated fats and cholesterol firm up the cell membranes, the omega-6 and omega-3 oils help to maintain their flexibility so that nutrients can easily pass into the interior of the cell and wastes pass back out. They also produce hormone-like substances called prostaglandins which play an important role in orchestrating the immune response. Study after study has shown that omega-3 oils are extremely protective to the heart, and they are also good for the skin, and essential for proper brain development and functioning. A deficiency can negatively affect mood as well as learning skills and cognitive ability, contributing to attention deficit disorder (ADD) in children.[13]

However, polyunsaturates that have been extracted from their food sources are extremely prone to damage by light, heat, and oxygen, leading to the production of dangerous free radicals, rogue molecules that steal electrons from healthy ones, crippling or destroying them in the process. When free radicals attack lipids, the resulting damage is known as lipid peroxidation. Whether this occurs by overheating vegetable oils or by keeping them longer than their shelf life, it transforms the lipids from health-giving substances to highly dangerous ones.

Hydrogenation

Commercial oil manufacturers try to get around this problem in one of two ways: either they "refine" the oils, which effectively strips them of most of their nutritional value, while adding chemical contaminants, resulting in the mediocre and often dangerous products that line supermarket shelves; or they partially hydrogenate them. Hydrogenation is a process of artificial saturation that uses high heat, aided by heavy metal catalysts, and results in the formation of extremely toxic *trans* fatty acids — substances which are literally closer biochemically to plastic than to their original food source. The end product now has an indefinite shelf life, precisely because everything of value in the original oil has been destroyed, leaving behind a transformed substance that is unfit for human consumption. Partially hydrogenated oils are widely used in the standard American diet, and are found in almost all fast foods, processed food, margarine, vegetable shortening, commercial baked goods, supermarket peanut butter, and movie theater popcorn. These fats literally gum up the cells of our bodies, and they are *directly* linked to clogged arteries, heart disease, obesity, diabetes, immune dysfunction, breast and prostate cancer, and many other degenerative conditions. As if that were not enough, they also sabotage the conversion of the healthy omega-6 and omega-3 oils into their biologically active forms, disrupt normal endocrine function, and interfere with the liver's detoxification capability.[14] Consider this next time you are tempted to head off with your children to your friendly, local fast-food restaurant for a meal of chicken nuggets and French fries, foods that deliver a whopping dose of these ultra-toxic altered fats! Unfortunately and inappropriately, they even show up in some items found in natural food stores, such as cookies, pies, and non-dairy "cheeses." Get into the habit of carefully reading the labels of all such goods, and avoid partially hydrogenated oils like the plague that they truly are. *Trans* fatty acids are the real villains in the fat wars, and they should be *completely* shunned by the health conscious consumer. They should be the proper target of the negativity unfairly directed at the naturally saturated fats.

The Omega-6 to Omega-3 Ratio

As we mentioned in Chapter 3, the ideal ratio between the natural omega-6 and omega-3 oils is between 4:1 and 2:1, whereas it is estimated that most Americans are getting somewhere between 10:1 and 20:1. An excess of omega-6 oils (corn, safflower, sunflower, and soybean oil) can have precisely the opposite effects than are achieved by the ideal ratio, producing pro- rather than anti-inflammatory substances that contribute to a host of degenerative diseases, while suppressing the body's ability to properly utilize the omega-3 oils. As omega-6 fatty acids are readily available in so many foods, using them as cooking and salad oils simply creates an unnecessary and destructive excess. Omega-3 oils, however, are much more scarce, being mainly found in cold-water fish (such as salmon, sardines, mackerel, and herring, all of which are Group II foods), and flax seeds (a food appropriate for both Groups I and II).

The unrefined oils used in Omega Nutrition's *Essential Balance Oil,* and other similar products such as *Udo's Choice,* are carefully processed to avoid damaging the delicate essential fatty acids. They are in a 1:1 ratio of omega-6 to omega-3 oils, based on the assumption that the additional omega-6 oils needed for the optimal balance with the omega-3 oils will be easily picked up through food. Approximately 50% is flax seed oil (yielding the omega-3 oil, alpha-linolenic acid), while the other 50% is a mixture of the predominantly omega-6 linoleic acid oils, sunflower, sesame, pumpkin, and borage oil. Borage oil (like the better known and more expensive evening primrose oil) contains a special omega-6 fatty acid called gamma-linolenic acid (GLA) that has similar anti-inflammatory properties to the omega-3 oils. However, due to the extreme fragility of these polyunsaturated oils, *Essential Balance Oil* must be refrigerated after opening, and must only be used cold. It is suggested that the Group I types—who require a lower fat intake than the Group II types—con-

RECOMMENDATIONS FOR USING OILS

∾ Use only unrefined, non-hydrogenated, preferably cold-pressed oils.

∾ Whenever possible, buy organic oils from crops grown without pesticides and herbicides.

∾ Use extra virgin olive oil as the preferred salad oil.

∾ For light cooking, use olive oil, sesame oil, or butter; unrefined coconut oil can also be used for any cooking purposes.

∾ Take care not to overheat oils; if an oil starts to smoke it should *immediately* be discarded and the kitchen thoroughly aired out.

∾ Take a 1:1 balanced omega-6/omega-3 oil daily as a food supplement, or use fish oils; do not heat these oils.

∾ Minimize the consumption of any additional omega-6 oils; get the balance of your omega-6 fatty acids from nuts, seeds, whole grains, avocados (for the Group II Metabolic Types), green leafy vegetables, or meats.

∾ Avoid all sources of partially hydrogenated oils, including margarine, vegetable shortening, fast foods, processed foods, commercial baked goods, supermarket peanut butter, and movie theater popcorn.

∾ Avoid French fries, chips that are not baked, and all deep-fried foods.

∾ Avoid refined supermarket vegetable oils (corn, safflower, sunflower, soy, canola).

∾ Buy oils in opaque containers that do not let in damaging light.

∾ Keep all oils and oil supplements refrigerated, except for coconut oil, and small amounts of olive oil that will be used up in a short period of time.

∾ Throw away any oil that has gone rancid, or that is past its pull-date.

sume one tablespoon daily of this oil blend, and that the Group II types consume two tablespoons. It can be used in salad dressings, added to yogurt or cottage cheese, blended into smoothies, or taken straight from the spoon. This simple practice alone can have profoundly positive ramifications for a person's health and well-being.

For some individuals, we recommend supplemental fish oils instead of plant oils, as people with cardiovascular problems, diabetes, or inflammatory conditions are often unable to convert alpha-linoleic acid into the active omega-3 fatty acids, EPA and DHA. Fish oils, unlike the plant-based omega-3 oils, are already in the form of EPA and DHA. No less than four recent reports in top medical journals further confirm the undisputed therapeutic properties of fish oils in particular, and omega-3 oils in general. In a long-term study published in *Circulation,* fish oils were shown to reduce by 45% the incidence of subsequent heart attacks in people who have already suffered one heart attack; in a study in *JAMA* (the *Journal of the American Medical Association*), women who ate fish five times a week cut in half their risk of fatal heart attacks, while women who only ate fish twice a month still lowered their risk by 20%; in the *New England Journal of Medicine,* men with high levels of omega-3 fatty acids in their blood were reported to be 81% less likely to die from fatal arrhythmias;[15] and in the *International Journal of Cancer,* a French study found an inverse correlation between levels of omega-3 fatty acids and breast cancer in women (that is, the higher the level of the omega-3s, the lower the occurrence of breast cancer).[16]

The Importance of Enzymes

Enzymes are often called the missing link to health, but what exactly *are* they? Enzymes are specialized proteins that serve as catalysts in biochemical reactions; in other words, they act as the spark plugs that ignite our metabolic motor. Our body produces thousands of different enzymes, each with particular functions that collectively are vital to every single metabolic process, including energy production, tissue growth and repair, the elimination of toxins, and the deactivation of harmful free radicals. Enzymes are essential to life itself, and without them, living organisms would perish.

Enzymes that are used for any purpose other than digestion are collectively referred to as metabolic enzymes. However, our pancreas also manufactures and secretes a special class of enzymes known as digestive enzymes, which are released into the small intestine following the ingestion of food and its initial processing by the stomach. Along with other enzymes secreted directly from the wall of the intestinal tract, these digestive enzymes help to break down our food into components that are small enough to be absorbed across the intestinal lining, where they are taken up by the blood and lymph systems to be distributed, via the liver, to the cells of the body. Like most enzymes, their names end in *-ase,* a suffix which is generally added to the root of the substance on which they act. For example, protease enzymes digest proteins, cellulase digest cellulose (plant fibers), lipase digest lipids (fats), lactase digest lactose (milk sugar), and amylase digests amylose and amylopectin (commonly known as starch).

Unfortunately, as we age the production of digestive enzymes tends to decline, and this is further exacerbated by the consumption of processed foods and excessive amounts of cooked foods. Research dating back to the 1930s shows that, when cooked food is ingested, the white blood cell count increases, indicating that the body is mounting an immune response.[17] This process, known as digestive leukocytosis, worsens if foods are pressure-cooked, and is most extreme with processed and refined foods, smoked meats, and microwaved foods.

Francis M. Pottenger Jr., M.D.—the son of the senior Francis M. Pottenger, M.D. who had earlier performed groundbreaking research into the autonomic nervous system—is well known for his famous cat experiments, which he conducted over several years, beginning in the early 1930s. He demonstrated conclusively that cats fed a raw meat diet lived long and healthy lives and produced healthy offspring, but that cats fed cooked meat developed various degenerative diseases, lived shorter lives, and produced progressively more unhealthy and short-lived litters.[18]

It is not entirely clear what the implications of this are for humans, as we have different digestive systems and metabolic needs than cats. All wild animals eat their foods raw. However, humans have been cooking at least some of their food for millennia. Certain foods, such as grains, beans, and the more fibrous vegetables, are virtually indigestible raw (unless sprouted), and require cooking to partially break down their fiber, making their nutrient content more readily available to the body. Cooking also reduces the possibility of potentially serious infection by such toxic organisms as salmonella, E. coli, and parasites. It also plays a key role in all the great cuisines of the world, and with its nurturing warmth and seductive fragrances, cooking adds to the pleasure of eating. It is well known that the simple enjoyment of food itself stimulates the activity of the digestive process.

However, we know that foods in their raw state come "prepackaged" with the enzymes needed for their own digestion. Unfortunately, these enzymes are easily destroyed by sustained exposure to temperatures above 118° Fahrenheit; thus, if we eat a diet that consists mainly of cooked foods, the entire burden of digestion is placed on our own pancreas. The pancreas seems to function best when it is assisted by the enzymes naturally present in raw foods, so a predominantly cooked food diet may tax the pancreas beyond its design limits, and may contribute to blood sugar problems, enlargement of the pancreas, and various degenerative diseases.

Thus it is wise to include at least some raw foods in the daily diet, to only lightly cook the more delicate vegetables (such as leafy greens), to use enzyme-rich fermented foods (such as yogurt or sauerkraut), and to supplement with digestive enzymes. Those on the Group I diet (Slow Oxidizers and Sympathetics) can generally handle a greater percentage of raw foods than those on the Group II diet (Fast Oxidizers and Parasympathetics), but some raw vegetables and fruits (as well as raw nuts and seeds, mainly for Group II types) are recommended for everyone. Raw animal foods are also used judiciously in most traditional cultures (steak tartare and sashimi being examples) but great care must be taken to minimize the possibility of bacterial or parasite contamination.

Supplemental enzymes are available from both animal and plant sources, and both contain the three main digestive enzymes: protease (to digest proteins); lipase (to digest fats); and amylase (to digest starches). Plant source enzymes generally also contain additional supportive enzymes, such as lactase, cellulase, maltase (to digest malt, produced in the breakdown of starches), and invertase or sucrase (to digest sucrose, or sugar). Animal source enzymes—usually derived from the pancreas of pigs, and referred to as pancreatin or pancreatic enzymes—are used mainly in therapeutic protocols, for which purpose they are taken between meals. This particular usage is most popular in Germany, where a proprietary blend of pancreatic and plant enzymes *(Wobenzym)* is the single best-selling, over-the-counter item sold in pharmacies. Plant source enzymes (such as those found in *Kristazyme;* see Resources) are primarily made from a special class of plant bacteria known as aspergillus, and are sometimes mixed with protein-digesting enzymes extracted from pineapple (bromelain) and papaya (papain). Plant source enzymes are the most useful daily supplemental digestive enzymes, and should optimally be taken at the beginning of a meal, or immediately before. They operate through a broad pH range (unlike animal enzymes), and (also unlike animal enzymes) work in the stomach as well as the small intestines, helping to break down our food and take the strain off the overworked pancreas. Because of the key role they play in releasing the nutrients from our food, digestive enzymes may be the most important supplement of all.

VITAMIN C AND THE METABOLIC TYPES

We all know that vitamin C is a powerful antioxidant that is vital to immune function and numerous other metabolic processes. As an essential nutrient (i.e. one that the body cannot make itself), it must be ingested daily from food or through supplementation. But are all forms of vitamin C appropriate for all individuals? From the perspective of Metabolic Typing, the answer is a resounding no! As we have seen, it is crucial that venous blood pH be maintained as close as possible to the ideal of 7.46. At this level, optimal absorption and utilization of nutrients can take place, whereas if the pH is too far off in either direction (below 7.46 would be too acid, above would be too alkaline), the ability to properly metabolize our nutrients will be compromised.

What is the Best Form of Vitamin C?

The two most common forms of supplemental vitamin C are ascorbic acid and calcium ascorbate (or other mineral ascorbates, such as magnesium/potassium/zinc/sodium ascorbate). *Ester-C,* a proprietary form of vitamin C often used in supplements, is a modified form of calcium ascorbate. Ascorbic acid is acid forming to the two Oxidative Metabolic Types (Fast and Slow Oxidizers). Fast Oxidizers already tend to have an overly acid blood pH, and so ascorbic acid—which would make them even *more* acidic— would not be an appropriate form of vitamin C for them. Conversely, Slow Oxidizers tend toward an overly alkaline blood pH, and so ascorbic acid helps to balance them out by making them more acidic.

Calcium ascorbate (and all the other mineral ascorbates, including *Ester-C*) is alkaline forming to the two Oxidative Metabolic Types. This would be a desirable effect for Fast Oxidizers (with their overly acid blood pH) but would be undesirable for Slow Oxidizers, who have an overly alkaline blood pH, and who would be pushed even further in the alkaline direction. Therefore calcium ascorbate helps balance out Fast Oxidizers, but would exacerbate the alkaline imbalance of Slow Oxidizers.

For the Autonomic Metabolic Types (Sympathetics and Parasympathetics), these values are reversed, because, as we have seen throughout this

Ascorbic acid *acidifies* the Oxidative Metabolic Types, which is:

- desirable for Slow Oxidizers (who are too alkaline);
- undesirable for Fast Oxidizers (who are already too acid).

Ascorbic acid *alkalizes* the Autonomic Metabolic Types, which is:

- desirable for Sympathetics (who are too acid);
- undesirable for Parasympathetics (who are already too alkaline).

Calcium ascorbate *alkalizes* the Oxidative Metabolic Types, which is:

- desirable for Fast Oxidizers (who are too acid);
- undesirable for Slow Oxidizers (who are already too alkaline).

Calcium ascorbate *acidifies* the Autonomic Metabolic Types, which is:

- desirable for Parasympathetics (who are too alkaline);
- undesirable for Sympathetics (who are already too acid).

book, nutrients that acidify the Oxidative types, alkalize the Autonomic types; and, conversely, nutrients that alkalize the Oxidative types, acidify the Autonomic types. Thus, ascorbic acid has an alkalizing (rather than acidifying) effect on the blood pH of the Autonomic types. This would be beneficial for the Sympathetics, who tend to have an overly acid blood pH; however, it would not be beneficial for the Parasympathetics, who already have an overly alkaline blood pH. Ascorbic acid would therefore further alkalize the Parasympathetics, and push them even more out of balance.

Calcium ascorbate, however, has an acidifying effect on both of the Autonomic types. This would create further imbalance in the Sympathetic types, whose blood is already too acid. However, it would help balance out the Parasympathetics, who need acid forming nutrients to counteract their overly alkaline blood pH.

The recommended form of vitamin C for the different Metabolic Types is as follows:

Group I
Ascorbic acid
Slow Oxidizers
Sympathetics

Group II
Calcium ascorbate
Fast Oxidizers
Parasympathetics

Thus, using vitamin C as an example, we can see how important it is to determine each individual's Metabolic Type. Such knowledge allows us to select the appropriate form of this vital nutrient, as well as *all* nutrients and foods, so that we can learn to intelligently and effectively balance our metabolism.

To C or Not to C

In March of 2000, the media trumpeted the results of a scientific study that appeared to imply that vitamin C supplementation might contribute to the hardening of the arteries. Naturally this has caused some concern among health-conscious consumers and clinicians alike, and has led many to leap to the conclusion that they should reduce, or even eliminate their vitamin C supplementation. But did the study in question—which was first reported in the *LA Times* before being picked up by the Associated Press—actually support this conclusion? The answer is a resounding no! The reporting of this study probably tells us more about the media than it does about vitamin C.

First of all, this study (which was conducted by a research team led by Professor James Dwyer at USC Medical School) used an imaging technology that is itself still undergoing trials for accuracy at the National Institutes of Health (NIH). Furthermore, the researchers only used one of the three indicators offered by this technology, a measurement for the thickening of the carotid artery. They did not use the other two parameters, one of which is a plaque index. Secondly, these data have yet to be peer reviewed, which is the standard evaluation process any scientific research must go through before it can even be published in a medical journal. Accordingly, it has not been accepted for publication in an accredited scientific journal. So, we have a study that uses only one of three indicators of a new technology of unverified reliability, that has not yet undergone the standard scientific review process.

But let us assume, for the sake of argument, that the research was indeed accurate. What then does it tell us? Essentially, it can be interpreted as a reminder of what we have known for years, that vitamin C strengthens arteries! This is one of the very reasons that nutritionists and holistic physicians have been urging people to take vitamin C all along! Where the confusion comes in is in the use of the term *thickening*. Thickening of the arteries is associated in the public's mind (and the mind of most physicians) with the hardening of the arteries that accompanies atherosclerosis, one of the most common precipitators of cardiovascular disease and heart attacks. Atherosclerosis is believed to result from injury to the lining of the arteries (caused by such factors as partially hydrogenated fats or elevated homocysteine levels), which in turn results in a buildup of plaque on the inside of the arteries. This plaque (composed, in part, of cholesterol and calcium) is actually a kind of "band-aid" intended to reinforce the weakened blood vessel, but it has the secondary effect of narrowing the inside of the artery, leading, over time, to occlusion (or clogging) and diminished blood flow to the organs.

If Professor Dwyer's study had demonstrated that vitamin C leads to occlusion, this would indeed have been a very serious and worrying conclusion. But this possibility was not even addressed by the study, nor is there a single shred of evidence from *any* other source to support this idea! However, this did not prevent the syndicated article publicizing its results from implying that it did indeed lead to such a conclusion. Whether this is simply irresponsible journalism or part of an ongoing strategy by the medical orthodoxy and the pharmaceutical industry (which provide the media with a substantial portion of its advertising revenue) to "discredit" vitamin supplementation is open to conjecture. The pharmaceutical industry is always looking for ways to undermine the value of nutritional supplements, as it (correctly) perceives them as a threat to huge drug company profits. Certainly the media knows that nothing sells like bad news! Much less attention gets paid to the veritable mountain of studies that continue to pile up, largely unheralded by the media, that show the *positive* benefits of vitamin C and other nutrients.

In fact, one of vitamin C's numerous virtues (it positively impacts almost every single metabolic process) is precisely that it helps the body to synthesize collagen, the connective tissue that is the basic building block of our blood vessels, tissues, and joints. As these tissues tend to thin with age, the thickening suggested by Professor Dwyer's study may well be very highly beneficial! Vitamin C is also a powerful antioxidant, working to destroy the free radicals that contribute to every degenerative disease that plagues our society—including heart disease.

Other news items in recent years have attacked vitamin C from other angles. In March 1998, a letter appeared in the prestigious scientific journal *Nature* from a team of British researchers, suggesting that vitamin C may, to some degree, act as an oxidant as well as the antioxidant that it is usually to assumed to be.[19] Oxidants unleash free radical attacks that can potentially result in DNA damage, a precursor the development of cancer; whereas antioxidants protect against these very processes. This was widely reported in the media as suggesting that vitamin C supplementation may actually *cause* cancer, even though the original letter never suggested this! Antioxidants, like vitamin C, are known to work in paradoxical ways, acting protectively (as antioxidants) in healthy cells, but destructively (as pro-oxidants) in unhealthy cells. In this way, they help the immune system to eliminate damaged cells, while protecting healthy ones. In response to criticism of their work, the authors of the original letter wrote a follow-up response in a later edition of *Nature,* in which they themselves stated that their own study indicated an overall protective effect of vitamin C.[20] Of course, this was not widely reported by the media.

Please do not be misled by these or any other media scare stories about one of the most valuable and highly studied of all nutrients. Instead, keep in mind a more recent article published in the world's most prestigious medical journal, *The Lancet,* showing that people who consume the most vitamin C in their diets have only half the death rate of people consuming the least. The most dramatic findings in this study, which tracked 19,000 men and women over a four year period, showed an amazing 93% fewer cases of heart disease deaths in women who consumed the most vitamin C, and 68% fewer in men. The men also exhibited a 53% lower risk of dying from cancer.[21] While it is true that the researchers were not studying supplemental vitamin C, but rather the vitamin C naturally contained in fruits and vegetables (yet another reason to eat plenty of them!), nevertheless the implications are still quite obvious.

The only real issue is how much vitamin C to take, and in what form. Many authorities argue that it is futile to take vitamin C in amounts exceeding 200–500 mg because of research findings suggesting that the body can only absorb this much at one time.[22] However, when spread out over the day (as usually occurs with multivitamin supplements), greater amounts can indeed be absorbed. Furthermore, the body's need for vitamin C goes up exponentially when it is under stress or combating any illness, whether it be the common cold or the flu, or a life-threatening infection or degenerative disease. Therapeutic doses of over 100,000 grams have been used by medical practitioners under certain circumstances,[23] though such high doses are not recommended without knowledgeable supervision. If too much vitamin C is ingested, the body will respond with temporary diarrhea. In fact, this phenomenon (known as titrating to bowel tolerance) can be used to determine an appropriate therapeutic dose during illness. So, keep taking your vitamin C—as ascorbic acid for Slow Oxidizers and Sympathetics, and as calcium ascorbate (or other mineral ascorbates) for Fast Oxidizers and Parasympathetics—and feel secure in the knowledge that you are taking one of the most versatile and protective of all nutrients.

THE NOT SO SWEET TRUTH ABOUT SUGAR

Sugar is one of those foods that we all know we should not eat, but we go ahead and eat it anyway! Dentists have generally done a good job of educating the public about the connection between sugar consumption and tooth decay, but in practice few people (including dentists themselves!) heed their warnings, beyond brushing and perhaps flossing their teeth. It is an undeniable fact that, as a race, we humans seem to possess a sweet tooth. Perhaps this stems from the fact that the first food human babies traditionally have consumed—their mother's milk—is itself relatively sweet (and also rich in fats and cholesterol, crucial for nourishing the infant's developing brain and nervous system); or perhaps it is an adaptive evolutionary trait that helped guide our early ancestors to relatively scarce wild fruits and vegetables that were full of vitamins, minerals, and phytonutrients (*phyto-* means plant). Whatever its origin, our sweet tooth has been inflamed by the increasing availability of refined sugar products over the last century.

When it was first introduced in the early nineteenth century, refined sugar was an expensive luxury item, and consumption was correspondingly low. Today, however, the average American eats a whopping 150 pounds of sugar per year, which roughly translates into 25 teaspoons per day, and may comprise as much as 20% of a person's total caloric intake! If you are wondering where all that sugar comes from, keep in mind that a single non-diet soft drink typically contains 10 or more teaspoons of sugar—and many teenagers (and adults, for that matter) drink several such sodas every day. (Diet sodas have their own problems, and also cannot be recommended.)

Furthermore, sugar appears in one form or another in almost all processed foods: in such obvious sources as cookies, candies, ice cream, breakfast cereals, and pastries; and in less obvious sources as muffins, salad dressings, sauces, canned or frozen vegetables, and smoked meats and fish, as well as many so-called "diet foods" and energy bars. (One very popular energy bar contains no less than eight different kinds of sugar, many of them going under names that the average consumer would not even recognize as sugar, and some of which FDA regulations do not require to be listed as "sugar" on the Nutrition Facts panel.) Sugar is even put in some brands of table salt, as well as in cigarettes, perhaps to add to the addictive power of the tobacco. In short, sugar is ubiquitous, and unless a person is eating a strictly whole foods diet, it is almost unavoidable.

So what exactly *is* sugar? There are many different kinds of sugar —most of their names end in *-ose* (such as glucose, maltose, and lactose) while others end in *-ol* (such as sorbitol and mannitol)—but the ones we consume the most are sucrose (table sugar) and fructose (mainly in the form of high fructose corn syrup). Refined from sugar cane or sugar beets, sucrose is a disaccharide (or double sugar) composed of one molecule each of the two most common monosaccharides (or simple sugars), glucose and fructose.

When consumed as a natural component of a whole food, sugar is metabolized fairly slowly due to the presence of fiber and various nutrient co-factors. But when eaten in its refined form, sugar rapidly enters the bloodstream, triggering the pancreas to release substantial quantities of the hormone insulin. Insulin, like all hormones, has many functions in the body, but one of its main ones is to usher glucose into the cells, where it is burned up in our cellular energy furnaces (the Krebs cycle of the mitochondria) to produce energy. This is what gives many people the familiar "sugar rush" or energy surge, while also stimulating the brain to release endorphins, our "feel-good" neurotransmitters.

If all this sounds desirable, we need to take a closer look at the problems associated with eating sugar. Most notoriously, regular sugar consumption plays havoc with our blood sugar levels. As the glucose rushes into the bloodstream, there is an initial glucose spike ("the sugar rush"), followed by a crash as the insulin clears it from the bloodstream to be burned up in the mitochondria. This leads to an energy slump, which tends to manifest as sleepiness, lethargy, and/or the desire to eat more sugar (or refined carbohydrates, which are simply composed of chains of glucose molecules) to bring our sugar levels back up. This yo-yo effect ends up stressing both the pancreas and the adrenal glands, which play a crucial role in overall stress and energy management. The adrenals have their own mechanism for dealing with low blood sugar, primarily by releasing adrenaline, which prompts the pancreas to release another hormone, glucagon; this in turn stimulates the release of glycogen, a starchy form of glucose that is stored in the liver and muscles as a short-term reserve fuel source to be converted back into glucose when blood sugar levels drop too low.

Hypoglycemia, or low blood sugar (*hypo-* is a prefix denoting under-functioning of a physiological system, gland, or organ), occurs when the blood sugar falls too low too quickly and the brain is deprived of glucose. The heart speeds up as adrenaline is pumped by the adrenal glands into the bloodstream, resulting in feelings that may include anxiety, shakiness, speediness, confusion, irritation, or depression. Fast Oxidizers are particularly vulnerable to this phenomenon, but it can affect any of the Metabolic Types if too much time passes without any food. Even if no symptoms are observed subjectively (as is commonly the case with Sympathetics who, like Fast Oxidizers, tend to burn up sugars and carbohydrates rapidly), low blood sugar is still a destructive phenomenon that should be avoided by eating regular meals.

Too much sugar (or refined carbohydrates) can also lead to the phenomenon of insulin resistance, where more insulin is produced than the cells can process. The result is that blood sugar levels remain elevated, leading to hyperglycemia, or high blood sugar. (*Hyper-* is a prefix denoting over-functioning of a physiological system, gland, or organ.) This is the primary hallmark of Syndrome X (see Chapter 4) and is also the precondition for Type II (adult onset) diabetes, a "disease of civilization" which is rampant in the U.S. today, and is increasing every year due to our collective infatuation with sugar and refined carbohydrates.

If glucose is produced in excess of our body's energy requirements, it turns into fat. This fat collects in the bloodstream in the form of triglycerides which, when elevated, are a primary risk factor for heart disease. Alternately, the excess triglycerides are stored in our adipose (body fat) tissues, paving the way for obesity. Furthermore, it has been known since the groundbreaking work of British researcher John Yudkin in the 1960s that eating sugar depresses immunity. Sugar impairs the activity of the white blood cells—our front-line defense against viruses and bacteria—for several hours after its consumption; as a result, people who eat a lot of sugar are more prone to catching colds and the flu.[24] (The term "catching a cold" or "a chill" relates a similar ability of cold weather to depress white blood cell activity, thereby rendering the chilled individual more susceptible to whatever viruses may happen to be present in their immediate environment).

Another problem with refined sugar is that it is also devoid of the very nutrients needed for its own metabolism, so it has to steal these from the body's own reserves. As such, it ends up depleting the body of nutrients, and can lead to deficiencies of B-vitamins and several important minerals, such as chromium. It can also interfere with the utilization of vitamin C (as both use the same transport mechanisms), as well as leaching calcium from the bones and teeth. Furthermore, it is known to raise blood pressure and triglycerides—both primary risk factors for heart disease—as well as contribute to arthritis and migraines. To add insult to injury, sugar is also the preferred food for bacteria and yeast, such as the potentially troublesome candida albicans, as well as for tumors, increasing the risk of breast and other cancers.[25] Some individuals are also flat-out sugar sensitive, meaning that their bodies react to sugar in much the same way that an alcoholic's body reacts to alcohol. Interestingly, often these individuals are children of alcoholics. For them sugar is truly an addictive substance. It powerfully modulates their brain chemistry, flooding them with the feel-good neurotransmitter beta-endorphin, leading to a physical and psychological dependence that is every bit as real as that produced by other addictive drugs.[26]

Sugar cane, from which much of our sugar is extracted, is a relatively benign food in its whole form, with a full complement of vitamins and minerals. The problems start with the refining process, which strips away almost all the nutrients, leaving behind pure sucrose. Most forms of "brown" sugar are simply white sugar that have been dyed with a little molasses, while "raw" sugar is simply a less refined version of white sugar that still retains some of its minerals. The two most benign forms of sugar are unsulphured black-strap molasses, which contains most of the minerals otherwise removed from white sugar, and evaporated sugar cane juice (such as *Rapadura)*, which is simply the evaporated juice of the entire sugar cane. Both of these forms of sugar are acceptable in small amounts, due to their high levels of nutrient co-factors, unless a person has an obvious blood sugar imbalance.

Artificial sweeteners like aspartame *(NutraSweet)* present serious health risks of their own. In fact, aspartame is a nerve toxin—probably due to the fact that it is processed using the very toxic methanol (wood alcohol)—and it generates the most complaints of any food substance to the Food and Drug Administration (FDA), ranging from headaches to seizures. Many people shun saccharin since it was reported to cause liver cancer in laboratory rats, although, humans bodies do not appear to contain the same enzyme present in rats that converts saccharin into its carcinogenic form. Nevertheless, it has absolutely no food value, and cannot be recommended, and questions still remain about whether or not it promotes cancer by some other means.

Fructose, which is commercially extracted from corn (and most commonly found in the form of high fructose corn syrup), has been touted as an alternative and healthier sweetener that does not spike the blood sugar as dramatically as sucrose. When naturally contained within a whole food, fructose (or any sugar, for that matter) is not likely to have negative effects, so long as it is eaten in moderation, due to the presence of fiber and the nutrient co-factors that help it to be properly metabolized; but when it is extracted and refined, fructose appears to be even more deleterious than table sugar. While it is true that it does not effect blood sugar as drastically as sucrose, it easily leads to the formation of advanced glycation end products (or AGEs). As we have already seen, these hybrid protein-sugar molecules are implicated in many degenerative diseases, including atherosclerosis and Alzheimer's disease, as well as in cataracts and the loss of skin tone. Animal studies further indicate that fructose may also raise serum triglycerides, as well as lactic and uric acid levels, and to generally accelerate the aging process.[27]

Fruit juices are also problematic, as they concentrate the sugars from the fruit while excluding the fiber that would otherwise slow down their absorption. Group II individuals (Fast Oxidizers and Parasympathetics) do best to avoid fruit juices entirely, and even the Group I types (Slow Oxidizers and Sympathetics) should only drink them in moderation, and preferably diluted or chased by a glass of water. Even carrot juice, a staple in natural food stores, packs quite a sugar punch. It is best used mixed with less sweet vegetables, such as celery or greens, and should also be consumed in moderation.

Other natural sweeteners —such as raw honey (cooked honey, which is the most common form, should be completely avoided), maple syrup, rice syrup, and fruit juice concentrates, as well as the aforementioned molasses and evaporated cane juice—will all tend to upset the blood sugar balance if used regularly, or in more than small quantities. However, because they contain some of the co-factor nutrients needed for their own metabolism, they are not as detrimental as the refined forms of sugar. Other sweeteners have also recently appeared, made of such exotic sources as agave (the same cactus from which tequila is made), kiwi, and a Chinese fruit called *lo han,* but not enough is known about them at this time to substantiate the claims made by their manufacturers that they do not significantly effect blood sugar levels.

Another new sugar is sucralose (marketed under the brand name *Splenda),* which is essentially regular table sugar (sucrose) with a molecule of chlorine added. The chlorine molecule is fairly successful in preventing the sugar from being absorbed, thereby avoiding an insulin response from the body, while the consumer still enjoys the sweet taste. However, not enough is known about any potentially deleterious effects of this substance, and chlorine itself is toxic. In tests on lab animals, negative effects were seen on the thymus, liver, and kidneys,[28] and although it is not known if it might have the same effects on humans, it would be prudent to minimize your consumption of this form of sugar until more is known about it.

Two natural sweeteners appear to offer unique benefits. The South American herb stevia *(Stevia rebaudiana)* is a small shrub in the chrysanthemum family that grows in the highlands of Paraguay and Brazil, where it is traditionally used to sweeten beverages, as well as for various therapeutic properties. Stevia contains steviosides and other glycosides, plant sugar molecules that, unlike other sugars, are not attached to carbohydrate substances. These lend stevia its sweetness which, depending on how it is processed, is anywhere from 15 to 300 times greater than sucrose![29] Stevia does have a distinctive taste, somewhat comparable to licorice, which some people enjoy, though others dislike it because it has a slightly bitter or "chemical" aftertaste. The best form of stevia to use is the ground leaf, which is available as a greenish-brown powder in the bulk section of many natural food stores. More refined versions are also available, either as granules in individual sachets or in liquid drops in small plastic bottles. Some recent research questions whether stevia may still elicit an insulin response (in the way sugar does), even though it appears not to directly effect blood sugar levels; probably the powdered leaf does so (if at all) less than the more refined versions.

The other sweetener with interesting properties is xylitol (pronounced "zy-lit-ol"), a natural sugar alcohol extracted from the fiber of birch tress, and also found in many fruits and vegetables, as well as synthesized by the body itself. Not only does xylitol *not* raise blood sugar and insulin levels, it also has numerous positive effects, including fighting plaque and the bacteria that cause dental cavities, helping to prevent infections (including ear infections in children), combating candida and other pathogenic yeasts, and nourishing the lining of the large intestine.[30] Xylitol, which contains 40% fewer calories than regular sugar, is not available in natural food stores at the time of this writing, but is available as a mail-order item. (See Resources for availability.)

For most of us, a little bit of sugar once in a while, though not recommended, is not going to have any serious effects, so long as we are eating an otherwise healthy, metabolically balanced diet. Stevia and xylitol are definitely the sweeteners of choice, while the other natural sweeteners can be used occasionally, and in moderation. We would suggest making sure you already have some protein in your system before you eat sugar, as protein helps to lessen its blood sugar spiking effects. (Parents, remember this for your children on Halloween!) But keep in mind that while a little bit of sugar probably will not hurt us, used regularly over many years it can indeed have truly disastrous health consequences, and can significantly contribute to many of the so-called diseases of aging. It is far better to stick to the proven benign sweeteners, stevia, and xylitol.

IN PRAISE OF EGGS
~

Eggs are one of the most underrated of all foods. In the 1970s and 1980s, eggs were subjected to an onslaught of attacks from the proponents of low-fat foods, who preached that they contained too high levels of the demon cholesterol to be fit for human consumption! Fortunately, the tides of nutritional opinion have turned, and the humble egg is once again being rehabilitated. Eggs contain an almost perfect amino acid profile. As we discussed elsewhere in this chapter, amino acids are the building blocks of protein (and, therefore, of our bodies), and eggs contain all the essential amino acids in almost perfect ratios, in a way that few other foods (except whey protein) do. As a result, the protein in eggs is exceptionally bio-available. Furthermore, eggs are an excellent source of vitamins A and D, the B-complex vitamins (especially folic acid and biotin), minerals such as calcium, potassium, phosphorus, and iron, and various types of lipids (fats), approximately two-thirds of which are unsaturated, and which include the essential fatty acids, omega-3 and omega-6. The whites are almost entirely composed of protein, while the yolks mainly contain the fats and other nutrients. Eggs also contain about 250 mg of cholesterol, which is the source of their undeserved infamy.

So what about cholesterol? First of all, cholesterol is—as we have previously mentioned—a vital nutrient, with numerous important functions: it gives strength to, and is a crucial component of, *all* the cell membranes in the body; it provides the raw material for *all* of the steroid hormones (including estrogen, progesterone, testosterone, and DHEA); it has antioxidant properties; is the precursor substance for vitamin D biosyntheis in the skin; is vital for the transport of fats and fat-soluble nutrients (such as vitamins A, D, E, and K) through the bloodstream to the cells; it is one of the main components of brain tissue; and it is essential to the proper growth and development of the nervous system of infants and young children, which is why it is found abundantly in human breast milk. Without adequate cholesterol in our bodies we would all die.

Fortunately, our liver manufactures its own supply, synthesizing approximately eight or more eggs' worth of cholesterol a day. So what happens when we eat cholesterol from dietary sources, such as eggs? The brain simply sends a message to the liver telling it to cut back on its production quota for that day. (A small percent of the population has lost this feedback mechanism, and so these few individuals may indeed need to limit their dietary cholesterol intake). Furthermore, eggs also contain a generous amount of lecithin, which helps to emulsify the cholesterol so that it flows freely through the veins without risk of clumping or oxidizing, while also conferring various brain-friendly properties of its own.

In the last few years it has become widely accepted that sugar, refined starches, and partially hydrogenated oils are the primary culprits that raise serum cholesterol levels, *not* dietary cholesterol itself. Additionally, other factors, such as elevated homocysteine, are now thought to be much more important than serum cholesterol levels in the development of atherosclerosis, the hardening of the arteries that is a major factor in many (but by no means all) cases of heart disease. (See Chapter 4 for more information on these risk factors.) Be that as it may, there has never been a single scientific study showing that eating eggs raises serum cholesterol levels to any significant degree, nor that eating eggs represents any increased risk of heart disease whatsoever! On the contrary, eggs have consistently been shown to be compatible with, and productive of, good health.[31]

Not all eggs are created equal, however. Commercially raised chickens eat an unnatural diet and live in concentration camp conditions that are not only inhumane but which require the use of antibiotics to control disease. The antibiotics end up in the eggs, and, therefore, the consumer. While antibiotics are valuable drugs in cases of severe infections, their indiscriminate use is implicated in breeding new, antibiotic-resistant "superbugs," as well as in the destruction of the important healthy bacteria (or flora) that normally reside in the human intestinal tract. The destruction of the benign intestinal flora leaves us wide open to colonization by opportunistic and pathogenic bacteria, viruses, fungi, yeasts (such as candida albicans), and parasites. (Antibiotics are also widely used in commercially reared, or non-organic beef and pork, as well as dairy cattle).

Furthermore, eggs produced in this fashion are nutritionally inferior, as indicated by their anemic pale yellow yolks. Health food store eggs (organic and/or "cage free") are considerably better in quality, but are generally not truly free range. Cage free chickens live in open-plan hen houses, under less crowded and more humane conditions than battery hens, but true free range eggs come from chickens that are free to peck around in the farmyard, exposed to sunlight, eating the seeds, greens, grit (for minerals), and bugs (yes, bugs!) that produce superior quality eggs. True free-range eggs are often found in local farmers' markets and, occasionally, in select stores. Incidentally, the color of an egg's shell has no bearing on its nutritional content. Many people assume that a brown egg is superior to a white egg (as brown rice is superior to white rice), but they simply come from different breeds of chickens.

Recently, a new type of egg has made its appearance, the omega-3 or DHA egg. You will recall from our discussion of fatty acids that DHA (docosahexaenoic acid) is one of the most metabolically active of the omega-3 essential fatty acids (it should not be confused with the similarly named hormone DHEA). These eggs generally come from cage free (but not free range) chickens, fed a special diet that includes foods such as flax meal that are high in the important omega-3 essential fatty acids; this gives the eggs a significantly higher omega-3 profile (ranging from a generous 150–225 mg per egg) than they would otherwise be expected to have. DHA is essential for the health of the brain, the nervous system, the heart, and the retina of the eye, and, while it is important for all humans, it is especially vital for infants and small children. DHA omega-3 eggs are also advertised to contain almost double the vitamin B-12 and up to six times the vitamin E of normal eggs. While free-range eggs may still represent the best choice, DHA omega-3 eggs and cage free, organic eggs represent good alternate choices. If none of these options are available, then regular commercial eggs would be the compromise choice. However, powdered eggs have been dangerously oxidized in processing, and are potentially quite harmful; they should be *completely* avoided. (Dietary cholesterol is only dangerous when it has been oxidized, which occurs as a result of the high heat used in the production of powdered eggs.)

Eggs are best eaten with the yolks intact (soft or hard boiled, or poached) to minimize oxidation of the fatty acids contained within the yolks. Scrambled eggs or omelets would be the next best choice, heated at the lowest temperature needed to cook the eggs. Fried eggs should generally be avoided, due to the damage caused both to the egg and the oil it is cooked in by the high heat involved. If you do want to fry eggs, use unrefined coconut oil (such as Omega Nutrition's *Coconut Oil*), as it is much more stable than other oils when heated, and cook the eggs slowly at a low temperature to avoid damaging their essential fatty acids. As long as the above caveats are observed, eggs are one of the most nutrient-dense foods on the planet, and happily are suitable for *all* Metabolic Types.

SOY RECONSIDERED

Everywhere you turn these days, health experts are touting the wonders of soybeans and soy products. We are told that they can do anything from preventing cancer to balancing the hormones of menopausal women. Soybeans do indeed have a long history of use in the Far East and are a good source of protein and other nutrients, but they are not without their problems and detractors.

Most of the soybeans currently being produced in the U.S. are genetically engineered, an issue which raises a whole series of disturbing questions in its own right. Despite the often compelling arguments advanced by the advocates of genetically modified (GM) foods (many of whom have a financial stake in their success), GM foods raise serious questions about potential long-term health risks which no one can as yet authoritatively answer. We simply do not have any meaningful data as to their long-term effects on the consumer and on the environment, and until more is known prudence would argue for erring on the side of caution. Additionally, soy is one of the most allergenic of foods, and its lectins (proteins that can lead to clumping of red blood cells) can potentially cause problems for people of all blood types, except, generally, people with blood Type O.

Part of the allergenicity problem may stem from the fact that soy contains protease enzyme inhibitors, which interfere with the body's ability to break down and assimilate its protein content. It is also exceptionally high in phytic acid (or phytate), a substance found to varying degrees in most legumes (and to a lesser extent in grains and nuts) that binds up zinc, calcium, iron, and other minerals, making it difficult for the body to absorb them. Certain foods do contain specific enzymes (known as phytases) which are able to break down the phytic acid, thereby releasing the minerals in its grasp; but at this time it is not certain whether or not these enzymes are normally found in the human intestinal tract. It is unclear, though, if this mineral blocking effect is significant in adults who eat plenty of other mineral rich foods; significantly, soy is usually eaten with mineral-rich seaweed in Japan. Interestingly, phytic acid (also known as inositol hexaphosphate) does have antioxidant properties, and it is even sold as a supplement (under the acronym IP-6) to help combat many ailments, including certain types of cancer.

To render soy more digestible, oriental cultures go to great lengths to prepare it properly. Soy milk and tofu (which is, essentially, coagulated soy milk) are thoroughly processed to reduce these anti-nutrient components, but only fermentation accomplishes this effectively. Therefore, the most "user-friendly" forms of soy are the fermented forms: tempeh, miso, and tamari (traditionally prepared soy sauce). Another problem with soy is that it is potentially goiterogenic—meaning that it contains compounds that, if eaten in large quantities, can undermine the healthy functioning of the thyroid. These compounds are none other than the isoflavones that are soy's main claim to fame! Whether or not regular use of soy can actually induce hypothy-roidism in a healthy person is open to debate; however, both clinical and sub-clinical hypothyroidism are already such common health problems that caution is certainly warranted, particularly in cases where these imbalances are known to exist. It should be noted, though, that iodine-containing foods (such as fish and seaweed) counteract this goiterogenic effect; and that these foods are commonly eaten along with soy in traditional Asian diets.

So what about the isoflavones found in soy that are being so heavily pro-moted as anti-cancer agents and hormone balancers? Its main isoflavones are genistein and daidzein and, to a lesser extent, glycetein. Isoflavones are a class of phytochemicals (plant nutrients) that have mild estrogenic, or estrogen mimicking, properties, and are therefore often referred to by the misleading term phytoestrogens (plant estrogens). It should be pointed out, though, that soy does not actually *contain* any estrogen, nor does it contain substances that the body can convert into estrogen. The so-called phytoe-strogens in soy and other plant sources are actually estrogen mimics and estrogen blockers—that is, they occupy the estrogen receptor sites in our cells, thereby partially preventing the body's own much stronger estrogens (particularly estrone and estradiol) from occupying these same sites. Accord-ing to the prevailing theory, the positive benefits of the weaker estrogen, estriol, are thereby received, as the isoflavones mimic the more benign actions of estrogen, while its undesirable effects (such as tumor promotion) are blocked.

Several studies have pointed to the cancer protective effects of isoflavones, particularly against breast cancer in pre-menopausal women. However, much less attention has been paid to the studies showing that isoflavones may actu-ally *promote* breast cancer in post-menopausal women, and pre-menopausal women with a previous history of breast cancer.[32] At this point the data are mixed, and women in these two risk categories might want to consider min-imizing or avoiding the use of soy products. An alternative is flax seeds, either eaten whole or ground into flax meal, and whole grain rye products, as these foods contain a type of phytoestrogenic fiber known as lignan which has demonstrated protective properties against cancer formation.

There are also concerns about the use of soy products in infant formu-las. Soy infant formulas contain levels of phytoestrogens that some researchers claim deliver a dose of estrogenic activity equal to several birth control pills.[33]

It is feared that this high level of estrogen mimicry might seriously interfere with the normal hormonal development in children, effecting maturation and fertility rates. However, this claim is disputed by other researchers who insist that the medical literature provides no evidence of untoward endocrine effects in children who are fed soy infant formulas. However, when this concern is combined with the potential mineral and protein blocking agents in soy (which may be more of a problem in a growing child than in an adult), caution would indeed seem to be advised. A spirited back-and-forth debate on this and other soy-related issues has been raging in the letters' column of the *Townsend Letter for Doctors* for over a year since the publication of a lengthy anti-soy article by two of its leading critics.[34]

Part of the problem here seems to lie in dosage. We in the West tend to believe that if a little of something is good for you, then more of it is even better, but this is often not the case. For example, while too little selenium in the diet greatly increases your risk of cancer (and as little as 200 mcg per day can significantly help prevent it), too much (which is, admittedly, rare and usually is the result of industrial contamination) can itself *cause* cancer. Soy protein powders, isoflavone supplements, and infant formulas often deliver concentrated levels of isoflavones never found in traditional Asian diets. Furthermore, many of the prepared food items that are made with soy (such as textured vegetable protein, soy "meats," soy cheese, etc.) are as highly processed as any other refined foods, and cannot therefore be legitimately considered as whole foods. For those whose systems do tolerate soy well, the fermented versions (tempeh, miso, and tamari) and smaller amounts of tofu and soy milk would appear to be the preferred forms. But soy eaten several times a day, or in large quantities, is almost certainly not advisable for anyone.

CHAPTER 7

Dental Toxicity

Early in my career as a dentist, it became obvious to me that the health of the mouth in general, and the condition of the teeth in particular, had to be connected to the overall health of the body. While this may seem like simple common sense, it remains to this day a radical idea in the world of dentistry. Other than warning of the dangers of excess sugar consumption in causing dental caries, most dentists (and certainly their professional dental organizations) do not proceed to make the logical connection between dental health and nutrition. I was fortunate in that my meeting with Adelle Davis, as recounted in Chapter 1, alerted me to the importance of nutrition. From then on I sought newer and better ways to incorporate nutritional work into my dental practice, and I began to devote one day each week to nutritional counseling for my dental patients. I explored numerous ways of assessing the state of the health of the body, particularly focusing on urinalysis, as the urine offers an easily accessible window into the complex world of our own biochemistry. Over time this work led me to discover George Watson's research into the Oxidative system, and I used this model for about ten years before Bill Wolcott introduced me to the integrated system of Metabolic Typing that we have been exploring in this book. When I decided to retire from my dental practice, I devoted myself to my nutritional work, in what was originally intended to be a part-time endeavor, which has since blossomed into a full-time preoccupation.

During the course of my dental career I also became aware of the toxic nature of many of the procedures that we dentists and our patients normally take for granted. I am indebted to the pioneering and courageous work of several leaders in this field, including George Meinig, D.D.S., Hal Huggins, D.D.S., and my long-time friend Doug Cook, D.D.S. To varying degrees these men have had to fend off less-than-good-natured challenges from their more closed-minded colleagues and the very conventional state dental boards and national organizations. It often comes as a shock to lay people to hear that many health problems can be caused inadvertently by traditional dentistry. What I am about to discuss will probably be new to many readers, although some may already have some knowledge on this subject. We will be discussing toxic metals, such as mercury and nickel, oral galvanism, possible toxic effects from root canals, cavitational problems from previous extraction sites, fluoridation, and the role of acupuncture in dentistry.

MERCURY AND NICKEL TOXICITY

A "silver" amalgam composition, or filling, consists of almost 50% mercury and 50% silver filings, to which small and varying amounts of tin, copper, and zinc may be added. The two main substances are triturated, or mixed together, into a mass that hardens in a short period of time. The widespread use of silver amalgams started in the mid 1800s. Since that time there has been an ongoing controversy about the toxic nature of mercury, and the appropriateness of its use as a dental restorative material. Because of growing public awareness of its dangers, the use of mercury for industrial purposes has waned. It is interesting to note that G. Agricola (in *De Re Metallica*) warned of the dangers of mercury pollution as long ago as 1556.[1]

Dental toxicity from mercury has been a highly inflammatory issue for the last 150 years. In fact, the term "quackery"—which is often indiscriminately applied to alternative health practitioners by their more conventional counterparts—was originally used in the nineteenth century to describe dentists who used the new silver amalgams, to the amazement of their more rational colleagues who were well aware of their dangers. However, the quacks took over the newly formed American Dental Association (ADA), and their quackery became standard practice. It has been the contention of the American Dental Association (ADA) that once the amalgamation (or solidification of the amalgam) took place there could be no leakage of mercury vapors from the filling. However, a landmark research project led by C.W. Svare in 1981 succeeded in documenting the release of mercury vapors upon chewing.[2] Even this did not phase the ADA, and their revised contention is that the amount of leakage is so small it has no ill effects on the tissues of the body.

However, another landmark study was conducted by Vimy, Takahashi, and Lorscheider of the Faculty of Medicine at the University of Calgary, in Canada. They placed twelve radioactive isotope silver amalgam fillings in five ewes. Each sheep was mated, and both ewe and fetus were monitored. Absorption of mercury into the fetus commenced on day two after placement of the amalgams in the ewes. The highest concentrations of mercury in the adult sheep occurred in the kidney and liver, with substantial levels also present in the endocrine glands, oral tissues, stomach, and respiratory tract.[3] This research project has been hailed worldwide for its meticulous documentation of mercury transmission from dental amalgams to distant parts of the body, but the ADA still refuses to accept its validity.

In 1984, I conducted before-and-after immune panels on twenty-nine patients with mercury and nickel restorations. Not only did the immune panels improve in most of these cases after the removal of the mercury and nickel, but various symptomatic health problems also improved dramatically. My report on this study was published in three different alternative medicine journals.[4] I would like to discuss two of those cases.

The first was a sixteen-year-old boy with exostosis, an abnormal growth of the bone. His father explained that the young man needed to have surgical procedures to free up his legs and arms every six months; he also said that the doctors did not expect him to live past the age of twenty-one. After hearing one of my public lectures on the hazards of mercury fillings, the father asked me if there was any possibility that mercury could be affecting his son's condition. I told him that mercury typically lowers the lymphocyte (white blood cell) count, and this, in turn, reduces the levels of T-lymphocytes, special white blood cells produced in the lymph glands and activated by the thymus gland that are essential for the proper functioning of the immune system. I explained to him that having the mercury fillings replaced would almost certainly improve immune functioning, and that this could only be beneficial.

He brought his son to see me and, upon examination, we found eight relatively small mercury fillings. We had an immune panel test performed by ImmunoDiagnostic Laboratories (IDL), and this panel showed an extremely compromised immune system. We removed the eight mercury fillings and replaced them with composite restorations. Six months later, we ran another immune panel, and the change for the better was astronomical. The father called me a year later and told me that his son did not need any more surgeries, and he was doing just great; he called me again the following year to report on his son's continued progress. He told me that the young man would probably live to be eighty or ninety, just like the rest of us.

The results of his immune panel were as follows:

	Before Mercury Removal	After Mercury Removal
Total Lymphocytes	2146	3515
Total T-Cells	1759	2988
Total T4s	751	1933
Total T8s	944	1195

You do not need a degree in immunology to see the sizable increase in all these numbers after the removal of the mercury fillings. The T4s are helper cells, providing a supportive function for other immune cells, while the T8s are cytotoxic killer cells, which destroy damaged tissues. There should be roughly twice as many T4s as T8s, but in this situation it was reversed, with more T8s that T4s. The immune system weakness was due to a lack of T4s. This suggested an autoimmune problem, a situation characterized by an excess of one type of immune cell at the expense of another. The young man's disease condition completely reversed itself after the mercury fillings were replaced, a procedure which has to be performed with certain safety precautions (such as the use of dental dams and air extractors) to prevent the vaporized mercury from being absorbed though the mucous membranes of the mouth or through the nose. Unfortunately, most dentists are not aware of the need to take such precautions when removing amalgams, and do not do so.

The next patient was a forty-eight-year-old female who had had breast cancer and a subsequent mastectomy five years before. I discovered that she had seven nickel crowns in her mouth, so I explained to her that nickel was carcinogenic and suggested that they should be replaced with gold. She was agreeable to this, and an immune panel was taken, which revealed a compromised immune system. Six months after I replaced the nickel crowns with gold replacements, we ran another immune panel test.

	Before Nickel Removal	After Nickel Removal
Total Lymphocytes	2046	3450
Total T-Cells	1575	2691
Total T4s	1043	1518
Total T8s	572	1069

Her total immune system strengthened substantially after the nickel was removed. You will notice in this profile that the T8s nearly doubled, while the T4s increased by 50%. Diseases characterized by a low T8 count include cancer, multiple sclerosis (MS), and lupus. There is a very real possibility that if this patient had earlier had the stronger immune system shown in the second column, she might never have contracted cancer, or if she had, that her immune system might have been more effective in counteracting it.

I would like to describe two other immune system related case histories that were published in *The Journal of Prosthetic Dentistry* in the 1980s.[5] The first was a young lady in her early twenties with seven mercury amalgam fillings. An immune panel was conducted to check her T-lymphocyte count before the removal of any amalgams. The immune panel showed that 48% of her total lymphocytes were T-lymphocytes, whereas the optimal number should be 80%. The mercury fillings were removed and replaced with temporary plastic fillings. After waiting 30 days, another immune panel was taken. The T-lymphocyte count had gone up to 80%. Her dentist then embedded four small mercury fillings in the lower plastic restorations. *These fillings never even touched the tooth structure.* Another immune panel was run thirty days later, and the T- lymphocyte count had dropped down to 53%. All the temporary plastic and amalgam fillings were then removed, and permanent gold fillings were put in their place. Then, thirty days later, yet another immune panel was taken. This one showed that the T-lymphocyte count had once again climbed back up to 80%. This very powerful research, conducted by David Eggleston, D.D.S. of the University of Southern California, clearly shows that our immune system can indeed be negatively impacted by mercury fillings, and that the body is capable of reversing the compromised immunity once the mercury is removed.

Another interesting case history relates to a young lady who checked herself into a university hospital suffering from a kidney ailment. The doctors diagnosed her as having glomerulonephritis, a potentially fatal inflammation of the kidneys, which they termed idiopathic (of unknown cause) as they could not find the causative factor. As the weeks went by, her condition became worse. They discussed the possibility of a kidney transplant to keep her alive. One of the doctors suggested she should have an electromagnetic allergy test performed to see if an allergy might be responsible for her condition. She did indeed show a severe reaction to nickel, and was asked if she had had any dental work performed recently. She replied that she had had two porcelain-to-metal crowns put in six months ago. Sure enough, the metal under the porcelain turned out to be nickel. She immediately had the crowns removed, and seven days later the symptoms of her nephritis disappeared. A kidney transplant was not necessary and she totally recovered.[6] How often does this kind of situation occur in today's world? Until the profligate use of mercury and nickel is curtailed, scenarios like this will continue to baffle physicians and cause unnecessary suffering in those unfortunate enough to be sensitive to these toxic metals.

ORAL GALVANISM

Oral galvanism is the difference of electrical potential created by two or more dissimilar metals in the mouth, or even by a single metal that conflicts with the body's own bioelectrical currents. Other names for oral galvanism are galvanic mouth currents, "mouth battery," and metal tension fields. All regulating events in the human body are communicated by electrical charges. Therefore, any conflicting electrical charges that emanate from dissimilar metals in the oral cavity create an imbalance that can lead to pathogenicity. In other words, the electrical currents created by the metals used in fillings and root canals can conflict both with each other and with the body's own electrical system, leading to blockages and interferences in the body's own bioelectrical currents. We were not born with such galvanic charges in our mouths; they are purely artificial. Our immediate concern should be to identify the nature of this problem and to stop using incompatible metals in the mouth.

Further toxic fallout comes from the dissemination of non-precious metal ions (atoms that carry an electrical charge) to distant areas of the body. Various fluids in the mouth—saliva, bone fluid, and dentinal plasma—act as conductors for electrolytes (minerals that dissolve in a fluid medium into electrically charged ions). Whenever a non-precious metal post is placed in a root canal for reinforcement, or an amalgam buildup is installed, or a gold crown constructed as a final restoration, measurable electrical currents emanate from that tooth. This leads to a disruption of the body's own internal electrical currents, which in turn has a negative impact on the functioning of the immune system, rendering us more vulnerable to inflammation and infection elsewhere in the body. Imagine the foci of infection and toxicity that can indirectly result from this "battery effect" in the mouth, silently permeating the body, and causing untold damage and ill-health. This problem is exacerbated by using different metals in the mouth, as they cross-react with one another. For example, even more galvanic currents will be created if a gold crown is installed, followed by a non-precious metal partial (a removable bridge) that contacts this gold crown. Unfortunately the brain does not pick up and neutralize these currents in the mouth, and so the spiral continues. I would estimate that between four and five million Americans suffer from this scenario. Couple this with 50–60 million Americans running around with mercury amalgams, and another 20 million with porcelain-to-nickel crowns, and what do you have? The set-up for a lot of degenerative diseases in the making. It is far preferable for only one metal ever to be used in the mouth, gold being the most desirable choice as it does not readily oxidize.

You might ask why, if all I have discussed is true, why hasn't organized dentistry picked up on this? Perhaps the two biggest reasons, which are closely connected, are fear and money. The fear comes from the many possible lawsuits that might occur if organized dentistry finally admitted that mercury in amalgams and other dental metals were toxic to humans. The official dental organizations have defended that position for so long that an about-face might open up a can of worms. The other reason is money. A dentist with a spouse, three children, a home mortgage, two cars, a dog, and a cat has to have a steady income. If such dentists were to deviate from mainline policies and practices, they might be faced with the very real possibility of reprisals from the state dental board. The possibility of a costly lawsuit or the loss of one's license are very real threats, and such a scenario did indeed overtake several of my colleagues. It obviously behooves the enlightened spirit to be not so outwardly enlightened, for fear of such reprisals!

I myself understand this situation all too well. The dental board visited my office on three occasions warning me of my failure to abide by the code of ethics, due to my refusal to toe the conventional dental line. These were weightless claims that merely served as a subtle form of harassment. Later the American Medical Association (AMA) secretary visited me to inform me that I was practicing medicine without a license. He told me that the dental board had supplied the AMA with information about my nutritional testing protocols, and that the AMA had deemed that I was treating cancers, kidney disease, etc., which went beyond the scope of my dental license. In fact, this was totally erroneous, as I was simply offering nutritional advice to my dental patients, and my dental license did indeed authorize me to practice nutrition. They told me if I ceased performing nutritional testing, they would drop their plans for taking away my dental license. I could ill afford to lose my license at that time, so I agreed to stop practicing nutrition for three years. This enabled me to get my house in order to prepare for my retirement. When the three years were up, I once again started performing nutritional testing. At this point I no longer fear any reprisals, as I am now only practicing nutrition, not dentistry, and so my license to practice dentistry has become inconsequential. I tell you this story to reiterate how difficult it is to be an enlightened spirit in a structured, inflexible, and dogmatic profession. One would like to believe that the dispassionate spirit of scientific inquiry would govern such matters, but all too often entrenched power interests overpower the very scientific point of view that they were originally intended to uphold. To quote Albert Einstein: "Great spirits often encounter violent opposition from mediocre minds."

Where does organized dentistry stand today on the issue of oral galvanism? The ADA has a similar position to that which they take on mercury amalgams. Although the scientific literature abounds with references to the problems caused by galvanic currents in the mouth, the powers that be are content to sit on their hands in the hopes that these findings will somehow go away. It is difficult to fight city hall, so even with technological advances and our growing knowledge of the problems of toxicity, fewer and fewer dentists are opting to travel the enlightened path. The progressive, holistic (or biological) dentist is between a rock and a hard place, but ultimately you, the patient, are being short-changed.

Root Canals

Next we turn our attention to root canals as a possible source of toxicity. Approximately twenty five million Americans undergo root canal therapy every year in an effort to prevent the loss of teeth that have become abscessed. The root canal refers to the central portion of the tooth, a canal that houses the nerve and blood vessels. During a root canal procedure, the dentist endeavors to clean and sterilize this canal, and then fill it in with a sterile, non-toxic, inert material. This usually renders this tooth serviceable and no longer painful.

The bulk of the tooth is made up of dentin, a material harder than bone, which is laced with a very large number of dentinal tubules. These tubules, or tiny tubes, facilitate the circulation of lymphatic fluid from the central root canal through the dentin, and out though the cementum (the outer membrane encasing the root of the tooth below the gum line) to the bone and gum tissue outside of the tooth. This is a viable circulatory system designed to service the root canal itself, its nerve network, and the periodontal ligament (gum and bone tissue) surrounding the tooth. If the body chemistry is healthy, the lymphatic fluid flows properly from the root canal through the dentin to the surrounding tissue, creating an irrigation system that serves to prevent an accumulation of plaque from forming around the root of the tooth. However, if the body chemistry is imbalanced, then the circulation can reverse, with lymph flowing from the outside of the tooth, through the cementum, and into the inner root canal—rather than out from it. This prevents proper irrigation, leading to an accumulation of plaque.

There are many additional reasons for maintaining the integrity of the circulation in the dentinal tubules, but root canal therapy completely destroys this integrity by filling in the root canal and preventing the proper directional flow of the lymph. So what, then, happens to the non-circulating lymph trapped in these tubules? It becomes stagnant and toxic, leaching out septic poisons into the bloodstream through the porous cementum. Mercury amalgams are said to be like caskets in the body, and root canals like cadavers. They are dead organisms that only serve to add to the body's burden of toxicity. I do not recommend root canals for anyone. However, each individual has a right to own their decisions, and many people simply do not wish to opt for the alternative, to lose the tooth (which is, after all, part of their body) through extraction. I respect this point of view, but I think it is important always to discuss the potential consequences of this decision.

Another related area of discussion is whether the root canal filling actually succeeds in sterilizing the apical end, or tip, of the tooth. This is a debatable point, as there are so many lateral canals at the root of the tooth that can harbor bacteria that it is unlikely that a completely aseptic, or sterile, condition will exist. But, again, the acceptance of root canal therapy as a viable alternative to extraction is completely and wholeheartedly supported by organized dentistry. Dentist are considered to be in violation of the code of professional ethics if they speak out against root canal therapy. When I was a practicing dentist, I always let my patients make the decision for themselves after explaining all the pros and cons.

CAVITATIONAL LESIONS

The next and last area of dental toxicity I will be discussing is the problem of unhealed extraction sites. These are called neuralgia inducing cavitational osteonecrosis (NICO), or jawbone cavitations. These areas may be a source of pain, but they cannot always be seen on an x-ray. The cause of these lesions is difficult to pinpoint. It is believed that if infection follows an extraction, or if a dry socket occurs after an extraction, the likelihood of a NICO lesion occurring is more likely. Even though the surgical site appears normal, a problem can exist in the bone for years. When these areas are biopsied, the abnormal features of a NICO lesion are discovered. It is not understood why some of these lesions are painful while others are not.

Based on laboratory findings, one or more of the following factors contribute to NICO development: immune system dysfunction or deficiency; unusual microbial pathogens; reduced blood flow to the affected part of the jaw; lack of one of several intra-bony growth factors; and nerve dysfunction. NICO lesions can cause pain, from mild to severe in some people. Pain from these lesions can be referred, or transferred, to distant organs. They can even refer pain across the midline, from one side of the mouth to the other, giving a false impression as to the source of the pain. Obviously, the best treatment is prevention, and this is accomplished by the dentist properly cleaning the soft tissue attachment, scraping the bone, and irrigating the socket with a homeopathic remedy. Generally, once NICOs are pinpointed, they are surgically cleaned out and biopsied to confirm diagnosis. NICO lesions are very perplexing. Even after surgery, they can reappear years later. Many times after the removal of these lesions, trigeminal facial pain subsides. (The trigeminal nerves control facial movement and chewing, and trigeminal pain can manifest in various parts of the face.) Many dentists are not familiar with this problem, but most oral surgeons are.[7] In the last fifteen years of my practice of dentistry, I observed approximately twenty patients exhibiting NICO, so you can see that, while not especially common, they do pose a very real problem.

FLUORIDE

Many of you are familiar with the controversy concerning fluoride. "No other procedure in the history of medicine has been praised so highly nor at the same time condemned so thoroughly," states George L. Waldbott in his book *A Struggle With Titans*.[8] The pro-fluoride forces believe that the benefits outweigh the risks, and that those risks are so small at the levels to which most of us are exposed as to be insignificant.

However, in 1977, John A. Yiamouyiannis, Ph.D. presented to Congress a controversial study that found that people living in the nation's ten largest fluoridated cities suffered 15% more cancer than those living in the ten largest non-fluoridated areas. What is even more frightening is that William L. Marcus, a senior scientific advisor for the EPA's (Environmental Protection Agency) Drinking Water Program, recently stated that the committee report not only overlooked liver cancer incidence but also would have reported "some" or "clear" evidence of carcinogenicity, had they not buckled under to pressure from pro-fluoride groups.[9] After making this announcement, Dr. Marcus was given thirty days to leave his job—another sad but clear example of moneyed interests outweighing serious public health concerns.

As you may already have guessed, my own feelings run strongly against fluoride. Fluoride is a form of the mineral element fluorine that is quite toxic at anything above infinitesimal levels. Too many vital enzyme systems in our body are compromised by it, leading to possible complications with arthritis, gastric ulcers, atherosclerosis, kidney disorders, migraine headaches, and, of course, cancer. The debate continues, but the pro-fluoridation forces are slowly losing ground. As our technology becomes more sophisticated, its detrimental effects are becoming more evident. There is the possibility that the fluoride might prevent dental caries to a limited degree, but the price we have to pay healthwise is simply not worth it. The bottom line is I would not prescribe fluoride treatments for my children; I would vote against fluoridated water; and I would recommend drinking only purified, non-fluoridated water.

ACUPUNCTURE

The last topic I will be discussing in this chapter is the role of acupuncture in dentistry, even though it does not directly relate to our primary theme of dental toxicity. There are two types of acupuncture: the traditional Chinese form that uses very fine needles inserted into acupuncture points located along the meridians (the bioelectrical pathways that connect up to different organ systems in the body); and electro-acupuncture. Both accomplish the same function but electro-acupuncture uses special equipment that allows the practitioner to determine the degree of imbalance in any meridian, as well as to deliver a mild electrical impulse to the acupuncture point to help correct that imbalance. The uses of acupuncture in dentistry are many. Pain relief, anxiety control, anesthesia, speeding up of the healing process, and differential diagnosing are the principle reasons for its growing popularity among holistic dentists, though it does take a few years to become proficient in this modality. Traditional Chinese acupuncture is taught in colleges of oriental medicine and at some universities, but electro-acupuncture is only taught through specialized professional groups.

Electro-acupuncture was researched and developed about fifty years ago by Dr. Reinhardt Voll, a medical doctor from Germany. After curing himself of colon cancer using Chinese acupuncture, he concluded he could make an instrument that would ascribe an accurate electrical value to each meridian.

This is how the EAV (Electro-Acupuncture according to Voll) unit was born. It was serendipitous that he discovered that homeopathy could also be used in conjunction with the EAV to determine exact potencies. The use of electro-acupuncture is still in its infancy, but the discipline is so accurate that I believe that it will be universally adopted by the medical profession for diagnostic purposes in the coming decades. In dentistry, where pain and rapid healing are so important, acupuncture can be very beneficial. I still use electro-acupuncture in my nutritional practice, not for diagnostic purposes, but for quantifying my clients' progress as they balance out their blood pH. Needless to say, it is a blessing that acupuncture is becoming an ever more accepted part of our health delivery system, and I contend that it is only going to grow in popularity.

FREQUENTLY ASKED QUESTIONS ABOUT DENTAL TOXICITY

∽

Q. How do I know if I have electrical currents in my mouth?

A. Many dentists have galvanometers to test millivolts, microamps, and microwatts per second. It is very similar to the voltmeter used in regular electrical work, but much more sophisticated. There is a state-of-the-art instrument called *Pertec*, which provides reproducible readings and is user-friendly. (Please see Resources for availability of the *Pertec*.)

Q. I hear that a lot of people get sick from having their mercury fillings removed.

A. This can indeed happen because the mercury is vaporized as it is being drilled out of the tooth, allowing it easily to pass though the mucous membranes that line the mouth, or through the nose, thereby entering the bloodstream. Certain precautions (such as the use of dental dams and air extractors) need to be taken by the dentist to minimize the chance of this occurring. Before any amalgam or nickel fillings are removed, a complete nutritional work-up should ideally be performed. Balancing the body chemistry and fortifying it with proper antioxidants (such as vitamin C and *AOX/PLX*) and homeopathics is very desirable to prepare for this procedure. Some dentists also use intravenous vitamin C infusions during the actual procedure to provide additional protection. Generally, when these precautions are taken, it is unlikely you will have any problems afterwards.

Q. Is it necessary to have material compatibility tests performed?

A. There are certain materials that are toxic to everyone, such as mercury and nickel. These should definitely be avoided. It is my feeling that anyone who already has toxic metals in their teeth will tend to demonstrate negative reactions to many other materials to which they would ordinarily not be allergic. The average cost for the blood compatibility test is $300. If proper judgment is used in the selection of non-toxic materials, I feel the compatibility testing is unnecessary.

Q. How do you feel about implants?

A. I have negative feelings about implants, as they represent a toxic foci similar to root canals.

Q. You holistic dentists each have different ideas on ways of rebuilding the mouth. Who do I believe?

A. Get a second and third opinion. It is your mouth, so exercise your own judgment, and go with the treatment plan that makes the most sense to you, and the dentist who most inspires your confidence.

Q. I have a bad reaction every time I have a local anesthetic. Do you have any suggestions?

A. Usually, it is the epinephrine in the anesthetic that causes the reaction, but there are anesthetics available without epinephrine. Another precaution is to take the homeopathic remedy aconite (at 6x strength) the day before and the day of your appointment. This particular remedy allays anxiety and will make you feel more comfortable.

Q. How do I find a holistic dentist?

A. This can be very difficult. Ask your friends if they know of any. Keep in mind that it is difficult for these enlightened spirits to practice openly, for the reasons I already mentioned. Please refer to the Resources section for the names of several organizations that can assist you.

CHAPTER 8

The End Is the Beginning

After reading through this book you will have arrived at certain conclusions about this new concept of Personalized Metabolic Nutrition, or Metabolic Typing. I hope it will be clear to you by now how this approach can have long-lasting benefits for your own health. Several decades ago, the late, great biochemist Roger Williams, Ph.D. introduced the concept of biochemical individuality into the lexicon of nutritional science, and, ever since it has become increasingly well established that every one of us is unique in our biochemical makeup. But within that uniqueness certain patterns of commonalty emerge that we refer to as the Metabolic Types. Based on the results of Metabolic Typing, a nutritional program can be initiated that can have the potential for bringing about significant and lasting changes in a person's health and well-being. It is estimated that it takes approximately fifty years for a new scientific finding to gain widespread acceptance; let us hope that Metabolic Typing will be embraced by the mainstream scientific community in a much shorter time than that.

The most confounding enigma in our work is why certain foods acidify the blood of one individual but alkalize the blood of another. George Watson, Ph.D painstakingly explained in his out-of-print classic, *Nutrition and Your Mind,* how the process of oxidation renders certain foods acid forming and others alkaline forming. This occurs through the biochemical transmutations that nutrients undergo as they are processed through the Krebs cycle inside our cells. Even more perplexing is how the very *same* foods that alkalize the Oxidative types (Fast and Slow Oxidizers) *acidify* the Autonomic types (Sympathetics and Parasympathetics), and how foods that acidify the Oxidative types *alkalize* the Autonomic types. When I first observed this phenomenon in one of my patients, it was a truly enlightening experience! While much is now understood about the role of the Krebs cycle in controlling the process of oxidation, less is known about autonomic dominance, or why foods have the opposite pH effect in the Autonomic types as they do in the Oxidative types. Nonetheless, this empirical finding represents a monumental breakthrough in the practice of nutrition, as well as having significant implications for the practice of medicine. Addressing the acidity or alkalinity of an individual's blood is of paramount importance in promoting the successful outcome of any therapeutic protocol, whether it be nutritional or medical.

We all have preconceived ideas about health, but it is important both to keep an open mind with respect to new scientific data, as well as to view such data with a critical eye. I come from a traditional medical background that demands controlled double blind studies to validate empirical findings. Empiricism is the observation of clinical data, and the theoretical conclusions that are drawn from these observations. Sometimes the observations may be valid, but the conclusions based upon them may not be. At other times both the observations *and* the theoretical model may be accurate, but it might be challenging to confirm them scientifically, simply because not enough is known about the system in question. This is the situation with the autonomic pathway of energy production. We do not know *why* autonomic dominance leads to foods having opposite effects on blood pH than oxidative dominance, but we are certain, based on many years of empirical clinical experience, that this is indeed the case. For example, proteins and fats alkalize the Oxidative dominant types but acidify the Autonomic dominant types. Noting this phenomenon every day in my practice has validated it beyond a shadow of doubt in my own mind—an example of the empirical approach. However, we are still unable to offer a scientific explanation for this phenomenon. I hope that, as Metabolic Typing becomes more established, funds will be made available to conduct a rigorous scientific investigation of this enigma.

We are working with some of the same metabolic markers as traditional medicine. Blood pH, oxidation rates, sympathetic and parasympathetic interactions, blood pressure, glucose tolerance, respiratory rates, the interplay between oxygen and carbon dioxide—all of these are part and parcel of the traditional medical world view. There is no reason why the medical profession should be at odds with our protocols. They are simply not widely known or understood. My mission is to spread the word far and wide, and this book is a vehicle to do just that.

Good health is such an important commodity, and it should not be taken for granted. My brother-in-law confided to me on his deathbed that he would have gladly given up smoking if he had known earlier that it would have prevented the emphysema that was killing him prematurely. The lesson to be learned is to make lifestyle changes before it is too late. My own preoccupation with health is based on several similar experiences with friends, relatives, and clients. Please humor me if I tend to be a bit unforgiving of the individual who is unwilling to make healthful lifestyle changes in the face of disease, as I know full well what the consequences can be. I also know the rewards that come from helping to turn an individual's health around—to hear people say that they have more energy, have lost weight, have fewer allergies, experience more restful sleep, and are enjoying a greater sense of well-being.

Nutrition picks up the ball where traditional medicine falls short. So many health problems can be corrected, or at least greatly alleviated, simply by knowing which are the right foods and supplements for any given individual. From cancer to the common cold, there is no health condition that cannot benefit from the application of the principles of Metabolic Typing. As nutritionists we do, of course, focus on the central role that nutrition plays in a person's overall health and longevity. But stress and toxicity are both known to exert wide-ranging negative effects on the body. Diet alone may not always be entirely sufficient to fully regain metabolic balance in the face of ongoing emotional stress, or the onslaught of toxic chemicals from mercury fillings, environmental pollution, and the contamination of our food, water, and the very air we breathe. Overwhelming though these factors may seem to be, we are not helpless in cleaning up our act. We can choose to feed ourselves and our families wholesome organically grown food, drink pure water, have toxic dental work removed, and exert pressure on our elected officials to clean up the environment. We can also stay physically active, exercise regularly, and be sure to get plenty of rest and sleep. All of these simple activities are vital to good health. We also need to be sensible and to seek proper medical advice and intervention when necessary. Above all, we must strive to maintain a positive mental and emotional outlook on life. Even in the face of disease, we can develop strength from adversity. Love and happiness are their own rewards, but they also build strong immune systems. Our stay on earth is brief, so let us do what we can to enjoy it to the hilt, to savor each moment and each day, and to maximize our life experience through the cultivation of radiant health.

The title of this chapter, The End is the Beginning, is a phrase coined, in part, to point to the necessity of more research on Metabolic Typing. However much we know, there is always more that we do not know. It is inevitable that such research will come about, as Metabolic Typing represents the beginning of a new era in nutrition and medicine, one in which therapeutic protocols are specifically targeted to an individual's Metabolic Type. However, the end of this book is also the beginning of your own journey of discovery. My work—which is also my joy—has been to lay out a path for others to follow as they explore this fascinating new approach to nutrition, nutrition for the new millennium. Your work—and, I hope, your joy—is to walk that path in health, happiness, and harmony. May you be blessed as you embark on this wonderful journey of discovery.

Understanding the Testing Protocols of Metabolic Typing

Following are the imbalances that are assessed during an office visit with a practitioner of Metabolic Typing. (Note that the *Personalized Metabolic Nutrition Self-Test Kit* focuses on the two primary imbalances, but is only able to assess one of the secondary imbalances, the Acid/Alkaline imbalance). Each of these imbalances and their related testing protocols are discussed in some detail in this appendix.

Primary Imbalances
1. *Oxidative Imbalance:* Fast or Slow Oxidizer
2. *Autonomic Imbalance:* Sympathetic or Parasympathetic

Secondary Imbalances
1. *Acid/Alkaline Imbalance:* Acidosis or Alkalosis
2. *Electrolyte Imbalance:* Electrolyte Stress or Insufficiency
3. *Anabolic-Catabolic Imbalance:* Anabolic or Catabolic

Metabolic Testing Protocols

Metabolic Testing is conducted over a two-hour period, before which the individual must have fasted for a *minimum of six hours* prior to starting the tests. The Questionnaire and Medical History Form optimally should be filled out prior to the time of the appointment. There are four testing cycles spaced at specific intervals (the starting point, thirty minutes later, forty-five minutes after the end of the thirty-minute cycle, and twenty minutes after

Blood Tests
- Blood glucose levels
- ABO blood typing

Saliva Analysis
- Saliva pH

Urinalysis
- Urine pH
- Urochrome Test
- Specific gravity
- Chemical panel (leukocytes, nitrites, protein, glucose, ketones, urobilinogen, bilirubin, blood, hemoglobin)

Vital Signs
- Blood pressure
- Pulse
- Respiration rate
- Breath hold capacity

Subjective Tests
- Questionnaire(dietary/physical/ psychological)
- Three questions (sense of well-being/energy level/hunger level)

Secondary Tests
(performed selectively by some Metabolic Typing practitioners)
- Vitamin C level
- Sedimentation

the end of the forty-five-minute cycle). The tests conducted at the starting point establish a series of baseline readings, after which the client is given a modified glucose challenge drink. The results of the subsequent three test cycles are then compared to the baseline readings. The blood glucose test and the three questions are repeated at every test cycle, but the urine, saliva, vital signs, and respiration tests are performed at the first and fourth cycles only. In the following section we are going to explore the various testing protocols that are used during the two-and-a-half-hour period of a typical office visit. We will then look at how we interpret the data derived from these tests, in order to determine the individual's Metabolic Type.

The Baseline Readings

When clients arrive for their initial appointment, we retrieve their Questionnaire and Medical History Form, and then ask them to give us urine and saliva samples. After determining their weight and body fat percentage, we then take a series of blood pressure and pulse readings, and check their respiration rate (how many times they breathe in one minute) and breath hold-

Personalized Metabolic Testing Chart

Name_____ Sex_____ Age_____ Date_____

Street_____ City_____ State_____ Zip_____

Phone(_____)_____ Fax or cell(_____)_____ E-mail_____

Bloodtype_____ Height_____'_____" Weight_____Body fat%_____Ideal weight_____Cycle day_____

Health concerns_____

Time of test:	Glucose-Potassium Challenge					Protein Challenge	
	Start	+30 min	+45 min	+20 min		+45 min	+45 min
Respiration rate (14–18)							
Supine pulse(68–77)							
Standing pulse 1							
Standing pulse 2							
Standing pulse 3							
Supine blood pressure							
Standing blood pressure							
Breath hold (50–80)							
Q1: Sense of well-being?							
Q2: Energy level?							
Q3: Hunger feelings?							
Blood glucose(80 120 100)							
Saliva pH (7.0)							
Adjusted saliva pH							
Urine pH (6.0)							
Adjusted urine pH							
Urochrome (3–5)							
Urine specific gravity							

Adjustment for Urine & Saliva pH

-0.5	1.000
-0.5	1.001
-0.5	1.002
-0.4	1.003
-0.4	1.004
-0.4	1.005
-0.3	1.006
-0.3	1.007
-0.3	1.008
-0.2	1.009
-0.2	1.010
-0.2	1.011
-0.1	1.012
-0.1	1.013
-0.1	1.014
0.0	1.015
0.0	1.016
0.0	1.017
+0.1	1.018
+0.1	1.019
+0.1	1.020
+0.2	1.021
+0.2	1.022
+0.2	1.023
+0.3	1.024
+0.3	1.025
+0.3	1.026
+0.4	1.027
+0.4	1.028
+0.4	1.029
+0.5	1.030
+0.5	1.031
+0.5	1.032

Questionnaire test results	Part 1	
	Part 2	
	Part 3	

	Leukocyte	Nitrite	Protein	Glucose	Ketones	Uro	Bilirubin	Blood	Hemo
Urine test strip									

	Vit. C (1–3)	Sediment (<0.4–>0.6)	Indican (<4–>4)			
Special tests						

	Pupil size	Ears	Cough	Gag	Tearing	Sleep	Urination	Clotting
Physical characteristics								

© Personalized Metabolic Nutrition 2002

MTT101

FIGURE A-1

ing capacity (how long they can hold their breath). All these data are recorded in the appropriate places on the Personalized Metabolic Testing Chart. (See Figure A-1.) This is followed by the first in a series of four blood glucose readings, taken at specific timed intervals. We then administer the glucose challenge drink.

All of the data collected up to this point serve as baseline readings against which the results of all the subsequent test data are compared. As its name implies, the glucose challenge drink is intended to challenge the metabolism of the client, to push it one way or the other. How their body handles this drink—the speed at which they process the glucose, how it affects the various metabolic markers, and how they respond to its effects subjectively—gives us valuable information that is used to determine their Metabolic Type.

The Glucose Challenge

When clients consume the glucose challenge drink, they typically have been fasting six to twelve hours, which usually simply means that they have not eaten or drunk anything (except plain water) since dinner the night before. (In our clinic, we generally schedule all our appointments during the morning hours so clients do not need to fast any longer than necessary). The drink itself is a modified version of the much more invasive glucose challenge drink traditionally given by medical doctors to test for diabetes or hypoglycemia. Our "mini" glucose challenge contains approximately 44 grams of glucose (less than half of the amount used in the conventional glucose challenge drink) and 5 grams of cream of tartar, which yields approximately 1 gram (1000 mg) of potassium. This mixture is diluted in approximately 12 ounces of distilled or filtered water. Many people find, to their surprise, that this drink is not especially sweet, but rather has a pleasant lemony tartness or "tanginess" to it, with an undercurrent of sweetness. Both of its ingredients will affect the metabolism: the glucose stimulates the Oxidative system (primarily targeting the Oxidative types, the Fast and Slow Oxidizers); and the potassium stimulates the Autonomic system (primarily targeting the Autonomic types, the Sympathetics and Parasympathetics).

I modified this drink, which I have been using in my work since 1988, from the writings of George Watson, Ph.D., the father of the Oxidative System, who describes it in his groundbreaking book *Nutrition and Your Mind*.[1] The inclusion of the potassium was drawn from the earlier research of Francis M. Pottenger, M.D., the man who was primarily responsible for developing our understanding of the Autonomic system.

In addition to affecting all subsequent readings (saliva and urine pH, blood pressure and pulse, respiration rate, and breath holding capacity), the glucose challenge drink is also used to infer or indirectly test the pH—or relative acidity or alkalinity—of the blood. Directly testing blood pH is impractical, invasive and costly, as it involves drawing blood intravenously four times over a fourteen-hour period. I did directly test blood pH in this way several hundred times in the earlier years, but I discovered that it is much simpler and less time-consuming to use the readings given by a glucometer, a blood glucose meter designed for monitoring blood sugar levels.

Using a small drop of blood drawn virtually painlessly from a fingertip with a spring-loaded lancet, the initial blood glucose reading is taken immediately before the glucose challenge is administered. This is then used as a baseline against which to compare the following three readings, taken at subsequent thirty, forty-five, and twenty-minute intervals, respectively. How quickly or slowly the glucose is metabolized, or cleared from the bloodstream, allows us to infer the relative acidity or alkalinity of the blood. To determine this, we add together the results of the first two blood sugar readings, then divide that number by two (e.g. if the first two readings were 80 and 120: 80 + 120 = 200 ÷ 2 = 100). This gives us the median number—the number that is midway between the first and second numbers—against which we compare the third and fourth blood sugar readings. If the third and fourth readings stay above the median number (e.g., are greater than 100, in our example), this implies that the blood is running on the overly alkaline side. If, however, the third and fourth readings fall below the median number (e.g. are less than 100, in our example), this implies that the blood is running on the underly alkaline side, which, for the sake of reference, we refer to as acid (as it falls on the acid side of the ideal blood pH level of 7.46). This pH tendency is then noted on the Personalized Metabolic Analysis Chart (see Figure A–2), where it can also be represented as a graph (the Glucose Chart), with a horizontal line drawn through the median point.

As previously mentioned, *all* blood is somewhat alkaline, never varying much more than two tenths of a percent on either side of the ideal level of

7.46; we use the terms acid or alkaline in a relative sense, to indicate whether the blood is on the overly acid side (or downside) or overly alkaline side (or upside) of this ideal. While the glucometer does not show us the actual pH of the blood, it does allow us to chart the tendency of the individual to run on the acid or alkaline side, which is all that needs to be known for the purposes of Metabolic Typing. The relative pH of the blood is directly linked to the speed at which a person clears the glucose from their bloodstream. Typically, people with acid blood (Fast Oxidizers and Sympathetics) clear glucose quite rapidly, with sugar levels often rising quite sharply (or "spiking"), then falling (or "crashing") equally sharply. By contrast, people with alkaline blood (Slow Oxidizers and Parasympathetics) exhibit a much less dramatic blood sugar curve, demonstrating a more gradual rise and fall of blood glucose levels.

Among the two acid types, Fast Oxidizers are usually very much aware of the roller-coaster ride provided by their spiking and crashing blood sugar levels, often becoming "speedy" or "wired" as the blood sugar spikes, then lightheaded, lethargic, sleepy, and/or increasingly hungry as it crashes; but Sympathetics are generally unaffected by such changes. Yet if we were to chart the Sympathetic's blood sugar curve on a graph, it might appear similar or even identical to that of the Fast Oxidizer. How, then, can it be that one of them is strongly affected by these blood sugar swings while the other remains oblivious to them?

The answer lies in the different dominance systems. The Fast Oxidizer's metabolism is directly controlled by the Oxidative system, the biochemical pathway that is responsible for the processing of the glucose in the mitochondria (or "energy furnaces") in the cells of the body; therefore, they are quite sensitive to fluctuations in blood sugar levels. The Sympathetic, by contrast, is controlled by the Autonomic system, especially the more *hyper* or energetic sympathetic branch of the autonomic nervous system (characterized by the well-known phrase, "fight or flight"). So, even though their blood sugar levels are being equally impacted by the workings of the Oxidative system, they are less affected by them because the Oxidative system is not primarily responsible for modulating their energy levels. Furthermore, the sympathetic branch of the nervous system is being directly balanced by the potassium in the glucose challenge drink, alkalizing the overly acidic Sympathetic type, and thereby providing the Sympathetic with sustained or even increasing energy levels. Thus, the Sympathetic is capable of being energized, at least for prolonged periods of time, solely by the action of the sympathetic branch of the autonomic nervous system.

Among the two alkaline types, the Slow Oxidizer typically responds to the glucose challenge with an equanimity similar to that of the Sympathetic; but the reason in this case is different. The Slow Oxidizer simply processes the glucose at a much slower pace than the two acid types (the Fast Oxidizer and the Sympathetic), and therefore does not experience the drastic blood sugar swings that afflict the Fast Oxidizer. However, the Parasympathetic tends to suffer similar negative reactions to the Fast Oxidizer, although generally not to the same degree. How can this be, given that the Parasympathetic is experiencing a gradual blood sugar response that is similar or identical to that of the Slow Oxidizer, who is largely unaffected by the glucose challenge?

Again, the answer lies in the action of the opposite dominance systems. The Parasympathetic (like the Sympathetic) is defined primarily by the action of the autonomic nervous system. Yet, while the Sympathetic draws on the more *hyper* branch of the autonomic nervous system, the Parasympathetic draws more on the *hypo*, or "laid back" branch of the autonomic nervous system (characterized by the phrase "rest and digest"). The potassium in the glucose drink heightens parasympathetic nervous system activity, and is alkaline forming in the Autonomic types. Thus, the Parasympathetic, who already runs on the alkaline side, is alkalized even further. Because the parasympathetic branch is more concerned with "resting and digesting," the result is that the Parasympathetic tends to lose energy, get sleepy or lethargic, and crave food to revive his or her flagging energy levels.

Charting the Test Results

Discovering the relative acidity or alkalinity of the individual's blood pH does not directly help us determine whether the individual is an Oxidative or Autonomic type, as there is an acid and alkaline type in both dominance systems. However, once we have determined the dominance system from our other markers, the blood pH does then allow us to narrow down which sub-type within that particular dominance system best characterizes the individual. So, first we determine the dominance system (Oxidative or Autonomic), then we determine the sub-type (Fast/Slow Oxidizer, or Sympathetic/Parasympathetic) within that dominance system. We will return to this part of the metabolic equation later on.

Whether an individual is Oxidative or Autonomic is primarily determined by how the glucose challenge drink affects the various other metabolic markers, between the first (baseline) and the second round of readings (which are taken shortly before the fourth, and final, blood glucose sample) — whether the saliva and urine have become more acid or alkaline; and whether the blood pressure, pulse, respiration rate, and breath holding capacity have increased or decreased. Typically, Oxidative and Autonomic types respond in opposite ways to all these parameters (as indicated by the plus and minus signs in the Autonomic/Oxidative section of the Personalized Metabolic Analysis Chart, shown on Figure A-2).

In both of the Oxidative types (Fast and Slow Oxidizers), the glucose challenge drink will typically *increase* the respiration rate, pulse, and blood pressure, but will *decrease* the breath holding capacity. Their saliva will become more acid, and their urine more alkaline. In both of the Autonomic types (Sympathetic and Parasympathetic), the glucose challenge drink will typically *decrease* the respiration rate, pulse, and blood pressure, but will *increase* the breath holding capacity. Their saliva will become more alkaline, and their urine more acid.

The Three Questions

In addition to evaluating these objective markers, we also factor in the client's subjective response to the glucose challenge. This information is gleaned from three questions, which are asked at each of the four testing cycles (i.e. each time a blood glucose sample is taken). The three questions, as asked at the first testing cycle, are:

1. "How would you rate your overall sense of well-being (i.e. how do you *feel*) *right now* on a scale of good, fair, and poor?"
2. "How would you rate your overall sense of physical energy *right now* on a scale of good, fair, and poor?"
3. "Are you hungry *right now?*"

The answers to these three questions are noted on the *Personalized Metabolic Testing Chart* with arrows: upward pointing (↑) for "good" (or "hun-

Personalized Metabolic Analysis Chart

Date_____

Name_____

Glucose Chart

Blood Glucose Level: 170, 160, 150, 140, 130, 120, 110, 100, 90, 80, 70, 60, 50

Time Start +30 +45 +20

Acidosis Alkalosis

	Glucose-Potassium Challenge		
	Acidosis	Alkalosis	
Respiration rate	≥19	≤13	Acidosis
Breath hold	≤40	≥65	Alkalosis

Autonomic/Oxidative

	Glucose-Potassium Challenge				Protein Challenge			
	Acid Blood		Alkaline Blood		Acid Blood		Alkaline Blood	
	Sym	Fast	Para	Slow	Sym	Fast	Para	Slow
Respiration rate change	−	+	−	+	+	−	+	−
Change in supine pulse	−	+	−	+	+	−	+	−
Supine diastolic b.p. Change	−	+	−	+	+	−	+	−
Breath hold change	+	−	+	−	−	+	−	+
Adjusted saliva pH change	+	−	+	−	−	+	−	+
Adjusted urine pH change	−	+	−	+	+	−	+	−
Change in well-being	↑	↓	↓	↑	↓	↑	↑	↓
Change in energy	↑	↓	↓	↑	↓	↑	↑	↓
Change in hunger	↓	↑	↑	↓	↑	↓	↓	↑
Totals								

Acid: severe / moderare / slight

Alkaline: slight / moderate / severe

Autonomic: Sym / Para

Oxidative: Fast / Slow

Electrolyte Imbalance

	Stress	Insuff
Highest pulse – lowest pulse	12+	12+
Supine systolic blood pressure	131+	112−
Standing diastolic blood pressure	88+	72−
Supine pulse		70−
Totals		

Electrolyte Stress
Electrolyte Insufficiency

Anabolic/Catabolic Imbalance

	Anabolic	Catabolic
Urochrome	2−	6+
Adjusted urine pH	6.3+	6.1−
Urine specific gravity	1.011−	1.020+
Adjusted saliva pH	6.6−	6.8+
Totals		

Anabolic
Catabolic

constipation	diarrhea
polyuria	oliguria
somnolence	insomnia

Questionnaire Results

Part 1		
Part 2		
Part 3		

MTA 101

FIGURE A-2

gry" for the third question), double-headed (↕) for "fair" (or "somewhat hungry"), and downward pointing (↓) for "poor" (or "not hungry").

The three questions are modified slightly the second, third, and fourth time they are asked:

1. "Do you notice any change in your sense of well-being since last time I asked you?"
2. "Do you notice any change in your physical energy level since last time I asked you?"
3. "Are you any more or less hungry since last time I asked you?"

At the end of the test, the predominant shift (if any) in the answers to the three questions are noted on the Autonomic/Oxidative section of the Personalized Metabolic Analysis Chart (Figure A-2). If the sense of well-being increased or remained high throughout, we circle the upward pointing arrows; if it declined or remained poor throughout, we circle the downward pointing arrows; if it was "so-so" throughout, we circle *all* the arrows (up and down). Note that Sympathetics and Slow Oxidizers share the same configuration of arrows, and that Parasympathetics and Fast Oxidizers share the opposite configuration of arrows.

As discussed above, Sympathetics and Slow Oxidizers (whom we collectively refer to as Group I types) tend to see a maintenance or improvement of their sense of well-being and physical energy, and they do not get particularly hungry during the testing period. However, Parasympathetics and Fast Oxidizers (who we collectively refer to as Group II types) tend to experience decreased levels of well-being and energy, and increased hunger during the testing period.

The Questionnaire and Medical History Form

The information culled from the client's Questionnaire (which is a more elaborate version of the Self-Typing Questionnaire shown in Chapter 2) provides further clues as to their Metabolic Type. Group I types (Sympathetics and Slow Oxidizers) tend primarily to circle the answers in the left-hand column (the FALSE answers), while Group II types (Parasympathetics and Fast Oxidizers) tend primarily to circle the answers in the right-hand column (the TRUE answers). Our Medical History Form alerts us to a client's individual health concerns, as well as providing further metabolic clues, as certain disease conditions tend to be more characteristic of particular Metabolic Types.

Determining Oxidative or Autonomic Dominance

After the testing is completed, we transpose the readings for each of the metabolic markers from the Personalized Metabolic Testing Chart onto the Autonomic/Oxidative section of the Personalized Metabolic Analysis Chart (Figure A-2).

For example, if the respiration rate has *increased* between our baseline reading (shown in the "Start" column of the Personalized Metabolic Testing Chart) and the second reading (shown in the "+20 min." column of the Personalized Metabolic Testing Chart), we circle the plus signs (+), which fall under the Fast and Slow Oxidizer columns. If it has *decreased,* we circle the minus signs (-) in the Sympathetic and Parasympathetic columns. We always circle the plus or minus signs in *both* of the two columns in which they appear, because the movement up or down of any given marker will always characterize two different Metabolic Types. In our current example, increased respiration rate would characterize both of the Oxidative types (Fast and Slow Oxidizers), while decreased respiration rate would characterize both of the Autonomic types (Sympathetics and Parasympathetics).

(Note that we are *only* circling the plus and minus signs in the four columns of the Glucose-Potassium Challenge section. The Protein Challenge section—to the right of the Glucose-Potassium Challenge section—is *only* used in rare cases where we decide that the use of glucose is contraindicated. This primarily occurs with individuals who demonstrate unusually low or high fasting blood sugar levels, or who have a strong negative reaction to the glucose challenge. In such cases, those individuals would be given a protein challenge drink, instead of the glucose challenge. Because the protein drink affects the metabolism in precisely *opposite* ways to the glucose drink, the pluses, minuses, and arrows in this section are exactly the inverse, or mirror image, to the pluses, minuses and arrows in the Glucose-Potassium Challenge section).

After circling all the relevant pluses and minuses, we then circle the appropriate arrows, as described above in the section on the Three Questions. We have seen that the same pluses and minuses will *always* be circled in the columns of members of the same dominance system. For example, *both* Fast *and* Slow Oxidizer columns will have exactly the same pluses and minuses circled as each other. Similarly, *both* the Sympathetic *and* the Parasympathetic columns will have exactly the same pluses and minuses circled as each other. However, a divergence appears when it comes to the arrows. While members of the same dominance system share the *same* response to the various objective metabolic markers, they demonstrate *opposite* responses in their answers to the three questions. The reason for this (which was explained above in the Glucose Challenge section) is that their shared response is experienced positively by one member of each dominance system, but negatively by the other member. So, instead of dividing the four types along the lines of their dominance systems, the arrows divide them along the lines of Group I (Sympathetics and Slow Oxidizers) and Group II (Parasympathetics and Fast Oxidizers). In other words, Group I is comprised of the two Metabolic Types (one from each dominance system) that respond positively to the glucose challenge, while Group II (also one type from each dominance system) is comprised of the two Metabolic Types who respond negatively to it. So, when the appropriate arrows are circled, the same arrows will be circled in members of the same diet group, rather than members of the same dominance system. Thus, Sympathetics and Slow Oxidizers (Group I) share the same directional arrows, while Parasympathetics and Fast Oxidizers (Group II) share the opposite set of directional arrows.

These groups are organized around the kind of diet that is recommended for each of the Metabolic Types (see Chapter 3). Each of these two groups consists of the acid type from one of our dominance systems (the Oxidative *or* the Autonomic) along with the alkaline type from the other dominance system. Group I is comprised of Slow Oxidizers (the alkaline Oxidative type) and Sympathetics (the acid Autonomic type); Group II is comprised of Fast Oxidizers (the acid Oxidative type) and Parasympathetics (the alkaline Autonomic type).

Next we tally the number of circled markers in each column and write the totals at the bottom. The Metabolic Type will generally be one of the two highest numbers shown. To determine which of these two is the true Metabolic Type, we then compare these two types with: (a) the results of the Questionnaire (to verify whether the individual falls into Group I or Group II);

and (b) the relative pH of the blood (acid or alkaline). For example, let us say that all nine markers are circled in the Sympathetic column, zero in the Fast Oxidizer column, six in the Parasympathetic column, and three in the Slow Oxidizer column (see Sample Analysis Chart I, Figure A-3). This individual is clearly one of the Autonomic types (Sympathetic or Parasympathetic), but which? Looking at their Questionnaire results, we can see that Group I questions predominate (the FALSE answers, in the left-hand column), which suggests that this individual is indeed a Group I type. This is reinforced by checking their blood pH, which is running on the acid side. Because Sympathetics have acid blood (and Parasympathetics have alkaline blood), this individual must therefore be a Sympathetic type. The other acid blood type, the Fast Oxidizer, had a zero score in the Autonomic/Oxidative tally, so clearly it is not a contender.

The example shown is what we might call a classic or "pure" Sympathetic type. Often, however, the markers will be divided among the different dominance systems. For example we may end up with tallies of four in the Sympathetic column, five in the Fast Oxidizer column, five in the Parasympathetic

Autonomic/Oxidative	Glucose-Potassium Challenge			
	Acid Blood		Alkaline Blood	
	Sym	Fast	Para	Slow
Respiration rate change	⊖	+	⊖	+
Change in supine pulse	⊖	+	⊖	+
Supine diastolic b.p. Change	⊖	+	⊖	+
Breath hold change	⊕	–	⊕	–
Adjusted saliva pH change	⊕	–	⊕	–
Adjusted urine pH change	⊖	+	⊖	+
Change in well-being	⬆	↓	↓	⬆
	⬆	↓	↓	⬆
Change in hunger	⬇	↑	↑	⬇
Totals	9	0	6	3

FIGURE A-3
Sample
Analysis
Chart I
(Sympathetic)

FIGURE A-4
Sample
Analysis
Chart II
(Mixed
Markers)

Autonomic/Oxidative	Glucose-Potassium Challenge			
	Acid Blood		Alkaline Blood	
	Sym	Fast	Para	Slow
Respiration rate change	⊝ (circled)	+	⊝ (circled)	+
Change in supine pulse	⊝ (circled)	+	⊝ (circled)	+
Supine diastolic b.p. Change	−	⊕ (circled)	−	⊕ (circled)
Breath hold change	+	⊝ (circled)	+	⊝ (circled)
Adjusted saliva pH change	+	⊝ (circled)	+	⊝ (circled)
Adjusted urine pH change	⊝ (circled)	+	⊝ (circled)	+
Change in well-being	↑	↓ (circled)	↓ (circled)	↑
	↑ (circled)	↓	↓	↑ (circled)
Change in hunger	↓	↑ (circled)	↑ (circled)	↓
Totals	4	5	5	4

column, and four in the Slow Oxidizer column (see Sample Analysis Chart II, Figure A-4). In this case, even though the individual is showing a slight predominance of Group II (Parasympathetic and Fast Oxidizer) markers, there is only a one point variable between any of the four types. Cases like this call upon the skill of the practitioner to weigh the relative values of the different markers. It should also be said no one marker can ever be relied on alone, hence the use of several different markers. For example, this individual may show several of the signs of being a Fast Oxidizer (a Group II type), yet they answered the Questionnaire in a manner more typical of a Group I type. In such a case, the practitioner would most likely discount the Questionnaire—which is subjective, and therefore more prone to inaccuracies—in favor of the predominance of the more objective metabolic markers.

Based on the above analysis, we are able to recommend a diet and supplement plan to bring the metabolism back into balance. Metabolic imbalances—which are the underlying causes behind most diseases—result from improper diet, lack of exercise, stress, and toxicity. Correcting them will enable individuals to enjoy the healthy productive life that is their birthright.

Secondary Imbalances

You may have noticed when looking at the Personalized Metabolic Testing Chart and the Personalized Metabolic Analysis Chart that certain of the test data were not discussed in our previous section on the testing protocols. These data relate to what we refer to as secondary imbalances—imbalances which do not define an individual's Metabolic Type but which might call for individualized modifications of the recommended nutritional protocols.

Urine Test Strip

On the Personalized Metabolic Testing Chart (see Figure A-1) there is a section labeled *Urine Test Strip*. This is one of several urinalysis tests we perform, and it is intended to show us if there are any unusual biochemical imbalances or pathologies reflected in the urine. Urine is an excellent medium for evaluating overall biochemical function because of its close relationship to blood—urine is essentially blood that has had its hemoglobin, or red blood cell content, removed by the kidneys—and because it is the repository of waste products from numerous metabolic processes. We look to see if there are unusual levels of leukocytes (white blood cells), nitrites, protein, glucose, ketones, urobilinogen, bilirubin, blood, or hemoglobin. These various factors relate to such processes as immune system capacity, protein metabolism, and the functioning of the pancreas, liver, and kidneys. Our intent is not to diagnose any medical problems (which is the exclusive province of physicians), but merely to see if any imbalance exists that can be addressed nutritionally.

Special Tests

Also on the Personalized Metabolic Testing Chart are boxes to indicate the results of three other urine tests. *Vitamin C* checks to see if there is an adequate amount of this all-important vitamin in the individual's system, and/or if it is being properly metabolized. *Sediment* evaluates how well the client is breaking down their food, and *Indican* specifically examines how well protein is being digested. An elevated indican reading suggests one or more of the following scenarios: inadequate hydrochloric acid (HCl) in the stomach; an imbalance of the bacterial flora in the intestinal tract (dysbiosis); incompletely digested protein in the large intestine (putrefaction), which produces toxic waste products that can leach back into the bloodstream; or a build-up of waste material (plaquing) on the wall of the colon. Useful though these tests are, they not essential to Metabolic Typing, and are not performed by many Metabolic Typing practitioners.

Acidosis and Alkalosis

These two imbalances—which, like all the following secondary imbalances, are indicated on the Personalized Metabolic Analysis Chart (see Figure A-2)—refer to processes that primarily involve lung and kidney (or renal) function, and center around the relative amounts of oxygen (O_2) and carbon dioxide (CO_2) in the system. (See *Oxygen, Carbon Dioxide and the Krebs Cycle* in Chapter 1 for a fuller discussion of this issue.)

∽ *Alkalosis* correlates with *hyperventilation* (over-breathing, or too many breaths per minute), a condition characterized by an excess of oxygen (which is alkaline forming) and a lack of sufficient carbon dioxide (and its by-product, carbonic acid); in an attempt to compensate, the body slows down the breath rate to limit the intake of oxygen and to prevent the loss of too much carbon dioxide.

∽ *Acidosis* correlates with *hypoventilation* (under-breathing, or too few breaths per minute) resulting in an excess of carbon dioxide and its metabolite carbonic acid (both of which are acid forming), and a lack of sufficient oxygen; in an attempt to compensate, the body speeds up the breathing to increase the intake of oxygen and to expel the excess carbon dioxide.

In either scenario, the kidneys attempt to compensate by excreting alkaline or acid urine, respectively, in order to restore balance. These imbalances need to be corrected by the use of specific acidifying or alkalizing agents.

Anabolic and Catabolic Imbalances

Our understanding of anabolic and catabolic processes is based on the work of the late, great Romanian physician, Dr. Emanuel Revici. Anabolic processes are those which control the synthesis, repair, and regeneration of bodily tissues. Catabolic processes are those which control the breakdown or recy-cling of bodily tissues. Both are vital to proper metabolic functioning, and exist in a dynamic, polar relationship to each other. When these processes are in balance, the body functions in a state of self-regulating equilibrium, or homeostasis.

Anabolism and catabolism play a key role in the production of energy within each cell. This is connected to their control of the permeability of the cell membranes, which can be likened to "skin" surrounding each cell. Proper cell membrane permeability is a vital function which determines how effec-tively oxygen and nutrients needed for the generation of energy can be deliv-ered into the cells, and how efficiently waste materials (which are a by-product of the generation of energy) can be removed from them. Cell membranes are composed of a double layer (technically known as a bilayer) made up of chains of two different kinds of lipids, or fat-based substances: fatty acids (the building blocks of fats), which provide flexibility and selective perme-ability; and sterols (primarily cholesterol), which provide strength and sta-bility. The proper balance between these two substances is crucial for optimal cellular functioning, including the production of energy.

∾ If the body exhibits an *anabolic imbalance*, there is an excess buildup of sterol chains in the cell membranes, in effect "clogging" them or making them too rigid, so that the cells cannot properly "breathe" (a process referred to as cellular respiration). The efficient inflow of oxygen and nutrients, and the outflow of wastes, is thereby compromised.

∾ In a *catabolic imbalance*, there is an excess build-up of fatty acid chains, resulting in overly permeable (or "leaky") membranes. In this case, the cells are breathing too freely, with insufficient regulation being exerted over the inflow of nutrients and the outflow of wastes. This is a process akin to hyper-ventilation at the cellular level.

Either one of these processes needs to be corrected through appropriate targeted supplementation.

Electrolyte Stress and Insufficiency

Electrolytes are minerals that, when suspended in the conducting solutions of our bodily fluids, carry an electrical charge. Sodium, potassium, calcium, and magnesium all function as electrolytes. Electrolytes are able to conduct electricity because their mineral salts separate out into electrically polarized ions (atoms that carry either a positive or negative charge). Electrolytes are vital for almost all tissue and cell functions.

~ *Electrolyte stress* occurs when the body's fluids become overloaded with electrolytes, leading to "clumping," or a lack of dispersion, which places a stress on the cardiovascular system, contributing to hypertension (high blood pressure).

~ *Electrolyte insufficiency* occurs when there are not enough electrolytes in the bodily fluids to adequately perform their many metabolic functions, contributing to low energy states and ineffective metabolic functioning.

Either one of these imbalances, if not corrected, can lead to various conditions of ill-health. They can be addressed through nutritional adjustments.

A Medical Doctor Looks at Cancer and Metabolic Typing

BY DR. ETIENNE CALLEBOUT

I first came into contact with Metabolic Typing in the 1980s through Dr. William Donald Kelley's work with cancer patients. I was also intrigued by the fact that a prominent young physician who was sent out to investigate Dr. Kelley's work, in order to declare it quackery, not only came to the opposite conclusion but started a practice based entirely on Kelley's methods. This doctor, Nicholas Gonzalez, M.D., of New York City, is, at the time of this writing, conducting a formal clinical trial with pancreatic cancer patients, supervised by the National Institutes of Health, in collaboration with the National Cancer Institute and Columbia College of Physicians and Surgeons. I contacted Dr. Gonzalez several years ago to ask about the methodology of Kelley's work, as he had access to most of Dr. Kelley's files. Unfortunately, there was never any response. The thought occurred to me that the Metabolic Typing fraternity operated like a secret society, where the people who had worked with Dr. Kelley were reluctant to share their information, probably due to the persecution that Kelley had suffered at the hands of the medical orthodoxy.

Finally, however, I was able to get into contact with William L. Wolcott, who had worked closely with Dr. Kelley for many years, and subsequently I encountered Dr. Harold J. Kristal via his published articles. I am deeply indebted to both of them for their willingness to openly share their knowledge. I fondly remember the day I spent with Dr. Kristal at his office, in which he explained to me the relevance of his glucose testing protocol, and helped me to finally obtain a copy of Dr. George Watson's long out-of-print classic, *Nutrition and Your Mind.* Bill Wolcott will always stand out because of his insights into the Autonomic and Oxidative systems and his further developments of our understanding of them. Dr. Milo Siewert, who also used to work with Kelley and now lives in England, also has always displayed an openness rarely seen in the field.

It is my hope that the groundbreaking research of Dr. George Watson and his follower Dr. Rudolf Wiley will be repeated and expanded—that individual foods will be re-tested both for their effects on the pH of the blood (as per Watson and Wiley's earlier research) and also on several other blood parameters. Further research will also be needed to establish the different hierarchies of Metabolic Typing—in other words, in addition to determining the individual's Metabolic Type, how can we establish the relative importance of endocrine (hormonal) predominance, catabolic/anabolic states, and other overlapping regulating systems? I personally will be trying to evaluate these by using the following modalities:

❧ **Heart Rate Variability Monitor:** a Russian instrument used to measure the predominance of sympathetic and/or parasympathetic activity within the autonomic nervous system;

❧ **Thermography:** a computerized imaging system that, apart from other detailed information, can tell me which body systems are physiologically (or pathologically) in an overactive or underactive state;

❧ **Darkfield Microscopy:** a special type of microscope that uses blood samples to evaluate the viability of such metabolic functions as the immune and digestive systems;

❧ **Biological Terrain Analysis (BTA):** measurements of the pH, electrical resistance, and redox potential of body fluids, based on the system of the Frenchman Louis Claude Vincent.

I was exposed to these methods through the work of Dr. Rau (Switzerland), Dr. Klinghardt (Seattle, WA), Dr. Stoff (Tucson, AZ), Dr. J. Chan (Vancouver, BC), Dr. Jurasunas (Portugal), Dr. Sheidl (Germany), Dr. Kristal, Bill Wolcott, and many others. I also cannot forget the publisher and alternative health advocate Burton Goldberg (Tiburon, CA), who is always a mine of information, both in person and via his publications. I mention all the above not only because of my personal gratitude towards them, but so that you, the reader, may find out more about their work, if so interested.

So how do I use Metabolic Typing in my own work? I employ the methods described in this book, integrated at times with some of Bill Wolcott's own techniques, modified as needed according to the particular clinical situation. I tailor my dietary recommendations to emphasize foods that have a low glycemic value (i.e. that do not cause the blood sugar to rise very quickly), as cancer cells feed much more voraciously on sugars than do healthy cells. These foods also need to contain proven cancer-protective phytonutrients. I make the patient aware of the Group I and Group II foods, which, on the forms I use in my office, are color-coded according to their respective group. Then I proceed to indicate percentages and quantities of certain foods. When working with cancer patients, high starch foods (which are rapidly metabolized into glucose) are greatly reduced, or their absorption is intentionally slowed by additional fiber or certain oils, such as medium chain triglycerides (MCTs) or flax seed oil.

Unlike other programs, mine instructs my clients to eat nothing after 3 P.M., with the intention of inducing a hypoglycemic (low blood sugar) state, which deprives cancer cells of their favorite food (sugars). (This correlates with the more drastic insulin-induced low blood sugar therapies used in some clinics to treat cancerous conditions.) A demanding fourteen-day fast often precedes this dietary regimen, and frequently a monthly five-day liver flush is also prescribed. It is imperative that the fourteen-day fasts be broken properly, with a carefully designed program to transition back to solid foods. A patient with breast cancer that had metastasized to the kidney (which is very rare in my experience) broke her fast with pizza, and ended up on the operating table with acute abdominal pains. Amazingly, upon examination, she was told by her doctors that they could not find a trace of any tumors anywhere in her whole body. (She had been on a modified Group II diet before the fast). It was obviously very encouraging to hear about the disappearance of the malignancy, but her abdominal distress would have been avoided had she broken her fast as directed!

I also evaluate blood antioxidant status (glutathione peroxidase), the essential fatty acid content of the red blood cells (RBCs), and the detoxification capacity of the liver. A sweat analysis informs me about the mineral status, as well as mercury and other heavy metal toxicity, and the standard blood chemistry analysis provides information about protein, fat, and carbohydrate status. I also look for (and frequently find) past or present indications

of infections of the herpes family, suggesting that herpes has more importance than we have assumed up to now. Frequently the mineral analysis
reveals low zinc and magnesium, and elevated copper and mercury levels,
with higher nickel levels also becoming more and more common.

The status of the teeth is also very important for overall health. This was
originally documented by Weston A. Price, an American dentist who extensively traveled the world in the 1930s, noting the positive relationship between
dental and overall health among so-called primitive peoples eating their traditional diets, and the subsequent decline in health among those who adopted
refined foods. This connection has since been further explored by Dr. Issels
in Germany and Dr. George E. Meinig and others in the U.S. Researchers
such as these have pointed to the toxic effects not just of mercury fillings but
also of bacterial foci in root canals (i.e. bacteria that were inadvertently
trapped in the tooth during root canal surgery). When root canal material
from unhealthy people is injected into rabbits, the rabbits almost always
acquire the same, or a similar disease as the root canal donor! This astonishing research finding has, for some inexplicable reason, never been properly aired in the media.

I also try to shift the immune system from CD4 /TH2 to CD4/TH1 activity (CD4 is a category of white blood cells, or lymphocytes, composed of TH
or T Helper cells). TH1 cells support the immune system's lymphocytes and
cytokines in identifying diseased cells, whether they be malignant or infected
with viruses. Vaccine therapies are often used in this context. It is also important to look into the cellular electromagnetic environment, or the electrical
potential of our cell membranes, a treatment area that is often neglected.
Cancer cells have a lower cell membrane potential, and it is of paramount
importance to try to increase it, a complex issue that is beyond the scope of
this article.

I continue to be fascinated by the well-documented association between
mycobacteria (such as the tuberculosis bacterium) and lung conditions and/or
cancer. Dr. Virginia Livingston-Wheeler was instrumental in making us aware
of it in her research, although a lot of her vaccine therapies seem to have
been based on Japanese studies done previous to her work. Let us also not
forget the use of the BCG vaccine in bladder cancers and the recent development of the English vaccine SRL 172 (based on *Mycobacterium vaccae*)
which shifts the immune system. Additionally, there is the MRV (mixed

response vaccine) used by Dr. Pitard (an American ENT professor), who used it to cure his own non-Hodgkin's lymphoma after he was given only a few months to live. He refused all other therapies and did his homework, also using cimetidine *(Tagamet)*, indomethacin *(Indocid)*, and interferon, using conventional medicines in a very unconventional way. He died ten years later of another, unrelated cause! The use of digitoxin merits further attention, especially after a Scandinavian study indicated a much lower incidence of breast cancer recurrence in patients using this drug. Mycobacteria are also used in the recent development of US cancer vaccines, along with other ingredients. Up until the early 1990s only so-called alternative cancer practitioners were interested in vaccines, as they had been for half a century at least; but then, suddenly, all the major pharmaceutical companies have started trying to develop them in the last ten years. Previously, vaccines had been seen as commercially self-defeating, as eradicating an illness is detrimental to long-term profits for the drug companies!

On a more philosophical note, even if the magic bullet for cancer is found, my impression is that sooner or later—based on the observation of medical history—another type of disease will come into prominence. This only further underscores the need for more research into Metabolic Typing, in order to provide a sound basis for an internal bodily environment that is unfavorable to the development of disease in the first place.

I always contact the treating oncologist before starting these dietary programs to ensure there are not any conflicting medications, and so that both of us are informed about the different approaches being used. I do not use Metabolic Typing assessments if the patient is already undergoing chemotherapy or radiation, as the individual is generally weakened from the treatment. I am also very doubtful about being able to accurately evaluate their Metabolic Type under these circumstances, as all their blood parameters are obviously going to be out of balance. I am happy if they simply have a good appetite! In such cases I recommend a basically healthy diet, emphasizing foods that are as close to their natural form as possible ("fruitcakes do not grow on trees"!), accompanied by supplements which, while not overly immune-stimulating, do help protect the body from the deleterious side-effects of chemotherapy and radiation, while simultaneously enhancing their cancer-killing effects. For further information on this strategy, please refer to the studies by Dr. Ralph Moss on chemo and radiation therapy that are readily available at most book shops and on the Internet.

In addition to diet, I also recommend coffee enemas (or other types of enemas), liver flushes, and immuno-active substances which, in one way or another, create an internal environment that is inhospitable to the proliferation of cancer cells. These include oriental mushrooms (such as *Coriolus versicolor* and maitake); unpasteurized whey protein (which increases the levels of the crucial antioxidant glutathione in normal cells, while decreasing it in cancer cells); green food concentrates; enzymes; specific proprietary herbal formulations; oxygenation therapies (germanium sesquioxide, *Zell Oxygen, Micom,* etc.); thymus extracts; DHEA, if indicated; placenta therapy (VG 1000), based on the Russian Dr. Valentin Gavollo's work; squalene; colostrum; fever-inducing therapies; and supplements specific to the individual's Metabolic Type.

The supplements are given five days a week for three weeks (i.e. fifteen days per month), while the fourth week is reserved, when needed, for detox therapy. Supplements are usually taken orally, but some may be taken sublingually (under the tongue), transdermally (absorbed through the skin), or by injection. Some exciting new manufacturing procedures exist to reduce substances down to 0.2 microns, allowing for much easier absorption under the tongue. This bypasses the digestive system, which is invariably weakened and compromised in cancer patients, as reflected in stool analyses (which typically turn up some bacteria, fungus, or parasites, as well as indicating absorption, flora, and enzyme disturbances).

It is not the focus of this appendix to emphasize psychological approaches to cancer therapy, but this does not mean that they are not important. The studies of New York psychologist Lawrence Leshan have highlighted the fact that the conventional psychotherapies—i.e. "what is wrong with you, and what you can do about it"—are of no relevance in regard to cancer survival. What does actually make a difference is an approach emphasizing "what is right with you, and what you can do about it"! This is not about denial, but about stimulating the limbic system (the emotional brain) into secreting the necessary substances to maintain a healthier immune system. Even more of an eye-opener is that the immune system is suppressed by as much as 300% for five to six hours after expressing anger, even recalled anger as in a conventional psychotherapy session. Incidentally, Dr. Leshan was able to do a good chunk of his work thanks to Dr. Emanuel Revici, mentioned earlier in this book as the formulator of the anabolic/catabolic system.

Cancer cells are not entirely controlled by the immune system. They are able to cloak themselves (like the Romulan battleships in Star Trek!) so that the immune cells pass by without recognizing them. Furthermore, cancer cells have the same electrical charge as immune cells, thereby repelling rather than attracting them, and they have a greater internal pressure. As a result, it is quite difficult for the immune cells to get access to the cancer cells in order to attack them. Additionally, cancer cells are able to grow their own blood vessels to nourish themselves (a process known as angiogenesis) without any direct connection to the autonomic nervous system, unlike any other blood vessels in the body. As a result, the brain does not even recognize the presence of these new blood vessels.

Also, let us not forget that insects do not even have an immune system, yet they do not seem to get cancer even if exposed to powerful nuclear radiation. Apparently their genetic repair capabilities are of a rather superior nature, which hopefully will be studied more closely someday. The only person I knew of who had a keen interest in this subject was the late German physician Hans Nieper, but unfortunately he died one week before I was supposed to meet him.

It has been observed that most patients with solid tumors (breast, prostate, colon cancer, etc.) are Group I types (Slow Oxidizers and Sympathetics), and that people with non-solid cancers (lymphomas and leukemias), melanomas, and sarcomas are more commonly Group II types (Fast Oxidizers and Parasympathetics). In my own work I have not yet been able to confirm this with the non-solid tumors. But I have seen people with myeloma (a form of bone cancer) change from being very Fast Oxidizers to very Slow Oxidizers at an astonishing speed after stem cell therapy. They developed totally different food tastes and hunger patterns, persisting even eight months after the treatment. An interesting research project would be to investigate possible changes in Metabolic Type before and after organ transplants, especially if the Metabolic Type of the donor was known.

I also have seen more and more people over the years with non-Hodgkin's lymphomas (NHL), for which there seems to be no adequate explanation. It should also be noted that, epidemiologically speaking, hormone-dependent cancers (of the prostate, breast, uterus, etc.) and digestive tract tumors seem to be much more diet-related than the other tumors,—i.e. there seems to be a causal relationship or correlation between poor diet and these types of cancers. As of this time I do not know if these types of malignancy will, on average, respond better to diet-based therapies. Even though I am aware that the purpose of using therapeutic diets is to create an environment unfriendly to cancer, it is worth remembering the work of the Nobel Prize winner Dr. Prigogyne (from Brussels, Belgium), who asserted—if I have correctly interpreted him—that a shock is often needed to jolt the body out of an unhealthy status quo situation. Perhaps, therefore, it is worth considering giving, for a short period of time, exactly the *opposite* kind of diet than is required. I have not yet seen enough evidence to know if this is a correct application of this concept, but it does raise the question as to whether or not homeostasis (or equilibrium) is really our most desirable condition. Unfortunately, more often than not, only a shock wakes us up.

On a practical level, I have seen patients with metastasized prostrate cancer and high PSA levels stabilize for four years, with nearly undetectable PSA readings, treated with no other therapies than the ones described above. A breast cancer patient following these regimes—as well as galvano (electrical) therapy—saved her breast, and apart from a scar that is only detectable on an ultrasound, shows no sign that she has had cancer. Understandably, this has given her an amazing psychological boost. A lung cancer patient who should have died two and a half years ago is now opening a shop in Notting Hill (a popular London neighborhood made famous in a recent movie of the same name starring Julia Roberts and Hugh Grant). He had extensive mediastinal metastasis (cancer spreading in between the lungs) which totally disappeared, as verified by CAT scans, one year later. In another patient, seven brain metastases were sharply reduced (by 75%) with oxygen therapies. This patient is also on the SRL 172 vaccine. He admits that he has long periods where he does not follow the diet, and he only starts up again if he gets worse. *C'est la vie!* Then there is the case of the young woman with stage four cervical cancer (i.e. with general metastasis, including to the lungs) who has now completely recovered, with all scans and tumor markers that were previously positive now within the lower end of the normal reference range.

The problem is that few people are inclined to continue to stick to the diet and supplement regime after the improvement of their condition, understandable though this may be from a normal human perspective. However, the famous French Paradox—that there are fewer cases of cancer and car-diovascular diseases in the wine-growing areas of France—does seem to contradict some of the diet restrictions imposed on cancer patients, such as the avoidance of alcohol. This partly can be explained by the powerful anti-cancer substances (bioflavonoids such as resveratrol, quercitin, and the proan-thocyanidins) found in the grapes from which the wine is made. However, few studies seem to emphasize the fact that many French people still have their main meal at lunchtime, enjoy an afternoon siesta, and eat lots of garlic, olive oil, and fresh vegetables, and enjoy more than average sunshine. All these factors seem to contribute to enhanced health. So, depending on the situation, I do not mind when people in the recovery phase drink red wine (preferably at least an eight-year-old Bordeaux) or French champagne (grown on soil full of ortho-phosphoric acid). Please understand that I do not intend to encourage alcohol consumption, but if I can find something to recommend to people that they might enjoy, I will happily do so.

It is important to stress that no one yet has the full answer concerning cancer, and that *all* options should always be considered, especially surgery. Finally, with deference to the importance of maintaining a positive attitude during cancer treatment, my most important prescription of all may well be: *enjoy life!*

Dr. Etienne Callebout is a Belgian medical doctor living and practicing in London, England. Dr. Callebout specializes in the treatment of cancer, incorporating Meta-bolic Typing into his treatment plan. We wish to stress that the protocols described are <u>*not*</u> *intended to be used as a self-treatment regimen, and are recommended for use only under the guidance of a qualified physician or oncologist.*

Resources

Note: the organizations below are listed for informational purposes only; a listing does not necessarily represent an endorsement of the services or products offered.

To Order the Personalized Metabolic Nutrition Self-Test Kit

Personalized Metabolic Nutrition
(415) 257-3099
(415) 257-3519 (fax)
hkristal@bloodph.com
www.bloodph.com

To Locate a Metabolic Typing Practitioner

www.bloodph.com
click on *Metabolic Typing Health Professionals in Your Area*

hkristal@bloodph.com,
(415) 257-3099
(415) 257-3519 (fax)

To Order Metabolically Balanced Vitamin Supplements

Personalized Metabolic Nutrition (PMN)
(415) 257-3099
(415) 257-3519 (fax)
hkristal@bloodph.com
www.bloodph.com

Multivitamins
Formula One
Formula Two
Formula Three

Digestive Enzymes
Kristazyme

Miscellaneous Supplements
AOX/PLX
L-Carnitine
Vitamin C (Group I)
Vitamin C Complex (Group II)

Expanded Cholesterol Tests

Atherotech Inc.
(800) 719-9807
www.atherotech.com

Berkeley HeartLab Inc.
(800) 432-7889
www.bhlinc.com

LipoScience
(877) 547-6837
www.liposcience.com

Hormone Saliva Testing Labs

Aeron Life Cycles
(510) 729-0375
www.aeron.com

BioHealth Diagnostic
(800) 570-2000
www.biodia.com

Sabre Sciences
(888) 490-7300
www.sabresciences.com

ZRT Labs
(503) 466-2445
www.salivatest.com

Hormone Creams (Non-Prescription)

Sabre Sciences
(888) 490-7300
www.sabresciences.com

Springboard
(866) 882-6888
www.springboard4health.com

Vitamin Research Products
(800) 877-2447
www.vrp.com

Compounding Pharmacies

International Academy of Compounding Pharmacists (IACP)
(800) 927-4227
www.iacp.org

Professional Compounding Centers of America (PCCA)
(800) 331-2498
www.thecompounders.com

Women's International Pharmacy
(800) 279-5708
www.womeninternational.com

Holistic/Biological Dental Organizations and Equipment

American Academy of Biological Dentistry
(831) 659-5385

Dental Amalgam Mercury Syndrome (DAMS)
(505) 291-8239

Environmental Dental Association
(800) 388 8124

Holistic Dental Association (HDA)
(800) 388 8124

Pertec Galvanometer
(920) 842-2083

Alternative Cancer Therapies

Anti-Neoplaston Therapy
The Burzynski Clinic
Stanislaw Burzynski, M.D., Ph.D.
(713) 335-5697
www.cancermed.com

Insulin Potentiation Therapy (IPT)
Steven G. Ayre, M.D.
Contemporary Medicine Center
(630) 321-9010
www.contemporarymedicine.net
www.itpq.org

Pancreatic Enzyme Therapy
Nicholas J. Gonzalez, M.D.
(212) 213-3414
www.dr-gonzalez.com

Miscellaneous Organizations

American College for Advancement in Medicine (ACAM)
(800) 532-3688
www.acam.org
(referrals to holistic medical practitioners)

A Campaign for Real Milk
(202) 333-HEAL
www.RealMilk.com
(information on raw milk dairy products)

Cognitive Enhancement Research Institute (CERI)
(650) 321-2374
www.ceri.com
(information on cognitive enhancement research)

The Price-Pottenger Nutrition Foundation
(619) 574-7763
(information on traditional dietary practices)

The Prostate Awareness Foundation
(415) 675-5661
www.prostateawarenessfoundation.org
(information and support groups for men with prostate cancer)

Radiant Life
(888) 593-8333
www.4radiantlife.com
(products and resources for optimal health)

The Weston A. Price Foundation
(202) 333-HEAL
www.WestonAPrice.org
(information on traditional dietary practices and sustainable farming)

**Nutritional Supplements
(Miscellaneous)**

Life Extension Foundation
(800) 544-4440
www.LifeExtension.com

Nutricology
(800) 545-9960
www.nutricology.com
Vitamin Research Products
(800) 877-2447
www.vrp.com

Xylitol

Vitamin Research Products
(800) 877-2447
www.vrp.com

Glossary

5-Alpha-Reductase: an enzyme that converts testosterone into dihydrotestosterone (DHT).

Acetyl Coenzyme Acetate (acetyl CoA): a substance created from the breakdown of carbohydrates, fatty acids, and amino acids, that plays a key role in generating energy in the Krebs cycle.

Adaptogen: a botanical or herb that is capable of modulating or balancing physiological functioning , especially the ability to respond effectively to stress.

Advanced Glycation End Products (AGEs): hybrid protein-sugar molecules involved in many degenerative disease processes.

Adenosine Triphosphate (ATP): the form of energy produced via the Krebs cycle and the electron transport chain.

Adipose Tissue: body fat.

Adrenal Glands: endocrine glands that sit on top of the kidneys that produce steroid hormones.

Aerobic: a process that requires oxygen to function (e.g. the Krebs cycle).

Allergenic: capable of producing an allergic reaction in sensitive individuals.

Anabolic: the process of tissue synthesis and repair, or the synthesis of larger molecules from smaller ones.

Androgens: hormones that produce masculinizing effects.

Androgenic: the masculinizing action of an androgen.

Andropause: the male version of menopause, characterized by a reduction in testosterone levels.

Androstenedione/Androstenediol: steroid hormones that are precursors to testosterone.

Anaerobic: a process that does not require oxygen to function (e.g. glycolysis).

Antioxidants: molecules that donate electrons to free radicals to "quench" them, thereby halting or preventing their destruction of healthy tissues; examples include vitamins C and E, lipoic acid, CoQ10, the mineral selenium, and many botanical extracts.

Aromatase: an enzyme that converts testosterone into estrogen.

Autonomic: refers to the autonomic nervous system (ANS), the master regulator of all involuntary metabolic processes (i.e. processes not generally available to conscious control); the ANS has two branches, or divisions: the sympathetic (characterized by "fight or flight") and the parasympathetic (characterized by "rest and digest").

Autonomic System: the Metabolic Typing system governed by the autonomic nervous system (ANS), responsible for the regulation and control of energy; the Autonomic system contains two sub-types, the Sympathetic and the Parasympathetic.

Autonomic Type: one of two Metabolic Types (Sympathetic or Parasympathetic) governed by the Autonomic system.

B-Cells: white blood cells involved in antibody production.

Beta-Oxidation: the process that breaks down fats into ketones.

Bioflavonoids: a special class of plant nutrients with antioxidant properties.

Blood Lipids: a collective term referring to cholesterol and triglycerides as found in the blood.

Catabolic: the process of tissue breakdown, or the breakdown of larger molecules into smaller ones.

Catecholamines: neurotransmitters that cause excitation or stimulation, such as dopamine or adrenaline.

Coenzymes: compounds, mainly derived from vitamins, needed to activate certain enzymatic reactions.

Co-Factor: a nutrient that works synergistically with other nutrients.

Dominance Systems: the two primary control systems that regulate metabolic function, the Oxidative system and the Autonomic system; each dominance system contains two sub-types, Slow and Fast Oxidizers, and Sympathetics and Parasympathetics, respectively.

Dysbiosis: an imbalance in the flora, or bacteria, in the intestinal tract.

Dysglycemia: a dysfunction of normal blood sugar metabolism.

Electron Transport Chain: a sequence of biochemical reactions involving the addition and removal of electrons that completes the work of the Krebs cycle in producing energy (in the form of ATP).

Endocrine Glands: glands that secrete hormones.

Fast Oxidizer: one of two Metabolic Types governed by the Oxidative System; Fast Oxidizers have an acid blood pH (below 7.46), and tend to burn blood sugar (glucose) rapidly.

Free Radicals: unstable molecules, or oxidants, that steal electrons from other molecules, causing a cascade of damaging effects that can lead to degenerative changes within the body, unless they are "quenched" by antioxidants.

Glucagon: a hormone secreted by the pancreas that releases glycogen from storage, to be converted back into blood sugar.

Glutathione: a potent antioxidant produced within the body that is crucial to the liver's detoxification capacity.

Glycogen: a starchy form of glucose stored in the liver and muscles as a reserve fuel source.

Glycolysis: a secondary form of energy production using glucose but no oxygen; glycolysis produces approximately 10–20% of our energy, generating lactic acid as a waste product.

Gonadotrophins: hormones that act on the testes or ovaries (e.g. luteinizing hormone, or LH, and follicle stimulating hormone, or FSH).

Homocysteine: an amino acid metabolite which, if elevated, is a primary cardiovascular risk factor; homocysteine levels are controlled by vitamins B-6, B-12, and folic acid.

Hormones: compounds produced by the endocrine glands that act on other glands or organs remotely, in other parts of the body.

Hyper-: a prefix denoting over-functioning of a physiological system, gland, or organ.

Hyperglycemia: elevated levels of blood sugar.

Hyperinsulinemia: elevated levels of insulin.

Hypo-: a prefix denoting under-functioning of a physiological system, gland, or organ.

Hypoglycemia: low blood sugar.

Hypothalamus: an endocrine gland in the base of the brain that works closely with the pituitary gland to control the other endocrine glands in the body.

Hypothyroidism: low thyroid function.

Insulin: a hormone secreted by the pancreas that controls blood sugar levels.

Ketones: compounds produced by beta-oxidation from the breakdown of fats.

Krebs Cycle: a biochemical energy-generating process that occurs within the mitochondria of each cell in the body (except mature red blood cells); it is the primary metabolic process responsible for converting nutrients into energy (in the form of ATP); also known as the citric acid cycle.

Lipids: fats, fatty acids, and fatty compounds like cholesterol.

Macronutrients: a collective term referring to protein, fats, and carbohydrates.

Micronutrients: a collective term referring to vitamins and minerals.

Metabolic Type: one of four distinct metabolic patterns, or ways of producing and processing energy, identified through Metabolic Typing (Slow Oxidizer, Fast Oxidizer, Sympathetic, or Parasympathetic).

Metabolic Typing: a system that identifies the characteristic way in which an individual produces and process energy.

Metabolism: the sum total of all bioelectrical and biochemical reactions that take place in a cell or organism.

Metabolite: a compound produced by metabolic action from another compound.

Mitochondria: (singular: *mitochondrion*) microscopic organs, or organelles, within all of the cells of the body (except mature red blood cells) that are responsible for generating most of the body's energy, through the Krebs cycle and the electron transport chain; the mitochondria are often referred to, metaphorically, as the body's energy furnaces or power stations.

Natural Killer (NK) Cells: a type of immune cell that targets and destroys cancer cells and other pathogens.

Neurotransmitters: brain chemicals that send biochemical nerve signals.

Oncogene: a gene that promotes the growth of cancer.

Oxidation: the process of the biochemical conversion of a substance using oxygen as a catalyst in the removal of electrons; in the Krebs cycle, oxidation converts nutrients into energy (in the form of ATP), a process that lends its name to the Oxidative system; however, oxidation can also produce unstable and potentially destructive free radicals.

Oxidative System: the Metabolic Typing system governed by the oxidative process, responsible for the generation of energy; the Oxidative system contains two sub-types, Fast and Slow Oxidizers.

Oxidative Type: one of two Metabolic Types (Fast and Slow Oxidizers) governed by the Oxidative system, the system responsible for the generation of energy.

Parasympathetic: one of the two Metabolic Types governed by the Autonomic system; Parasympathetics are governed by the more relaxed ("rest and digest") branch of the autonomic nervous system (associated with the stomach, liver, pancreas, and intestines), and have an alkaline blood pH (above 7.46).

pH: an abbreviation of *potential of hydrogen,* pH is a measurement of acidity or alkalinity of a compound or system; the scale runs from 0, which is extremely acid, to 14, which is extremely alkaline; 7.0 is neutral; numbers below 7 are considered acid, and numbers above 7, alkaline; however, because the ideal venous blood pH is 7.46, which is slightly alkaline, for the purposes of Metabolic Typing, anything below 7.46 (rather than 7.0) is considered acid, and anything above 7.46 (rather than 7.0) is considered alkaline.

Phytochemicals/Phytonutrients: special nutrient compounds found in plants that are not categorized as vitamins or minerals.

Phytoestrogens: a special class of phytonutrients that have an estrogen-like effect in the body, such as soy isoflavones.

Pituitary: an endocrine gland in the base of the brain that secretes hormones that control many of the other endocrine glands in the body.

Slow Oxidizer: one of the two Metabolic Types governed by the Oxidative system; Slow Oxidizers tend to burn blood sugar (glucose) slowly, and have an alkaline blood pH (above 7.46).

Steroids: hormones produced in the adrenal glands, testes, and ovaries that are manufactured from cholesterol; the term also refers to potentially dangerous pharmaceutical drugs that are modeled after the body's own steroid hormones.

Sub-Clinical: a condition of metabolic imbalance that does not produce sufficient symptoms to warrant a formal medical diagnosis.

Sympathetic: one of the two Metabolic Types governed by the Autonomic System; Sympathetics are dominated by the more proactive ("fight or flight") branch of the autonomic nervous system (associated with the pituitary, thyroid, and adrenal glands), and have an acid blood pH (below 7.46).

T-Cells/T-Helper Cells/T-Lymphocytes: various white blood cells involved in immune function.

Xylitol: a plant sugar with antimicrobial properties.

Xenoestrogens: (pronounced "zeno-estrogens") industrial or agricultural chemicals found in the environment that have an estrogen-like effect in the body.

References

Chapter 1

1. Kristal, Harold J., D.D.S. "The Death of Allopathic Nutrition." Address to the Orthomolecular Health-Medicine Society. San Francisco, CA, March 1998.
2. Williams, Roger J. , Ph.D. *Nutrition Against Disease* (New York: Bantam Books, 1978).
3. Ornish, Dean, M.D. *Dr. Dean Ornish's Program for Reversing Heart Disease* (New York: Random House, 1990).
4. Atkins, Robert C., M.D. *Dr. Atkins' New Diet Revolution* (New York: WholeCare/Avon, 2001).
5. Barry Sears, Ph.D. and Bill Lawren. *The Zone* (New York: Harper Collins, 1995).
6. Simonton, O. Carl, M.D. *Getting Well Again* (New York: Bantam Books, 1978).
7. Pottenger, Francis M. Jr., M.D. *The Cat Studies* (San Diego: Price-Pottenger Nutrition Foundation, 1995).
8. Pottenger, Francis M., M.D. *Symptoms of Visceral Disease* (St. Louis: C.V. Mosby, 1944).
9. Watson, George, Ph.D. *Nutrition and Your Mind* (New York: Harper and Row, 1972).
10. Wiley, Rudolf, Ph.D. *BioBalance* (Hurricane, UT: Essential Science Publishing, 1998).
11. Watson, *op cit.*
12. Kelley, William Donald, D.D.S. *One Answer to Cancer* (Internet: Do-It-Yourself-Book, 1999).
13. Spector, Michael. "The Outlaw Doctor." *New Yorker* (76)45 (Feb. 2001):48–61.
14. Peat, Ray, Ph.D. "Altitude and Mortality." *Ray Peat's Newsletter* (June 2000):1–5.

Chapter 3

1. Wiley, Rudolf, Ph.D. *BioBalance.* (Hurricane: Essential Science Publishing, 1998).
2. Hattersley, Joseph G., M.A. "The Nearest Thing to a Perfect Food: Part II." *Townsend Letter for Doctors* 227(June 2002):86.
3. Ross, Julia, M.A. *The Diet Cure.* (New York: Viking, 1999).
4. Enig, Mary, Ph.D. *Know Your Fats.* (Silver Spring, MD: Bethesda Press, 2000).
5. Fallon, Sally. "Cancer Increase." *Wise Traditions* 2(4) (Winter 2001):13–14.
6. Rowen, Robert Jay, M.D. "New Fat Reduces Abdominal Fat." *Second Opinion* (February 2002):1–4.
7. Schmid, Ronald, N.D. *Traditional Foods Are Your Best Medicine* (Rochester: Healing Arts Press, 1997).
8. Hattersley, *op cit.*
9. Waldbott, George L. *A Struggle with Titans* (New York: Carlton Press, 1965).
10. Wolcott, William L. and Trish Fahey. *The Metabolic Typing Diet.* (New York, Doubleday, 2000).
11. Wiley, *op cit.*

12. Watson, George, Ph.D. *Nutrition and Your Mind* (New York: Harper and Row, 1972).

13. Kelley, William Donald, D.D.S. *One Answer to Cancer* (Internet: Do-It-Yourself-Book, 1999).

14. Young, Robert O., Ph.D. and Shelley Redford Young. *The pH Miracle* (New York: Warner Books, 2002).

15. De Vries, Jan. *10 Golden Rules for Good Health* (Edinburgh: Mainstream Publishing, 2001).

16. Wiley, *op cit.*

17. Sullivan, Krispin, C.N. *The Lectin Report* (www.krispin.com).

18. Pottenger, Francis M., M.D. *Symptoms of Visceral Disease* (St Louis: C.V. Mosby, 1944).

Chapter 4

1. Wolf, Naomi. *The Beauty Myth* (New York: Harper Trade, 2002).

2. Price, Weston A. *Nutrition and Physical Degeneration.* (San Diego: Price-Pottenger Nutrition Foundation, 1975).

3. Fallon, Sally, and Mary Enig, Ph.D. "What Causes Heart Disease." *Wise Traditions* 2(1) (Spring 2001):15.

4. Fallon, Sally. *Nourishing Traditions* (Washington, DC: New Trends, 1999).

5. Francis, Raymond. "Sugar: A Poor Choice." *Beyond Health News* (July/August 1998):4.

6. Atkins, Robert C., M.D. *Dr. Atkins' New Diet Revolution* (New York: WholeCare/Avon, 2001.

7. Schwarzbein, Diana, M.D. and Nancy Deville. *The Schwarzbein Principle* (Deerfield Beach, FL: HCI, 1999).

8. Eades, Michael R., MD. and Mary Dan Eades, M.D. *Protein Power* (New York: Bantam, 1996).

9. Eades, *op cit.*

10. Lee, John R., M.D., and Virginia Hopkins. *What Your Doctor May Not Tell You about Menopause* (New York: Warner Books, 1996).

11. Rosedale, Ronald, M.D. "Insulin and Its Metabolic Effects." Address to the Designs for Heath Institute BoulderFest, August 1999.

12. Shames, Richard L., M.D. *Thyroid Power: 10 Steps to Total Health* (New York: Quill/Harper Collins, 2002).

13. Störtebecker, Patrick, M.D., Ph.D. *Mercury Poisoning from Dental Amalgam* (Stockholm: Störtebecker Foundation, 1985).

14. Selye, Hans, M.D. *Stress Without Distress* (New York: Signet, 1974).

15. Wilson, James L., N.D., D.C., Ph.D. *Adrenal Fatigue: The 21st Century Stress Syndrome* (Petaluma: Smart Publications, 2001).

16. Reaven, Gerald M., M.D. *Syndrome X: The Silent Killer* (New York: Fireside/Simon and Schuster, 2000).

17. Rosedale, *op cit.*

18. Reaven, *op cit.*

19. Bernstein, Richard K., M.D. *Dr. Bernstein's Diabetes Solution* (New York: Little Brown, 1997).

20. Rosedale, Ronald, M.D. *The Fountain of Truth* (Asheville, NC: Tanner, 1999).

21. Reaven, *op cit.*

22. Reaven, *op cit.*

23. Atkins, *op cit.*

24. Sears, Barry, Ph.D. and Bill Lawren. *The Zone* (New York: Harper Collins, 1995).

25. Ornish, Dean, M.D. *Dr. Dean Ornish's Program for Reversing Heart Disease* (New York: Random House, 1990).

26. Reaven, *op cit.*

27. Rosedale, Ronald, M.D. "Insulin and Its Metabolic Effects." Address to the Designs for Heath Institute BoulderFest, August 1999.

28. Price, *op cit.*

29. Watson, George, Ph.D. *Nutrition and Your Mind* (New York: Harper and Row, 1972).

30. Bayan, Matthew J. *Eat Fat, Be Healthy* (New York: Fireside/Simon and Schuster, 2000).

31. Wayne, Howard, M.D. *How to Protect Your Heart from Your Doctor* (Santa Barbara: Capra Press, 1994).

32. Wilson, *op cit.*

33. Lee, John R., M.D., Jesse Hanley, M.D., and Virginia Hopkins. *What Your Doctor May Not Tell You About Premenopause* (New York: Warner Books, 1999).

34. Lee, John R., M.D., David Zava, Ph.D., and Virginia Hopkins. *What Your Doctor May Not Tell You about Breast Cancer* (New York: Warner Books, 2002).

35. Douglass, William Campbell, M.D. "Estrogen Fails to Protect the Heart, Causes Cancer." *Second Opinion* (April 2001):4–6.

36. Schenker, Guy R., D.C. *An Analytical System of Clinical Nutrition* (Mifflintown. PA: Nutri-Spec, 1999).

37. Douglass, *op cit.*

38. Goldberg, Burton. *Alternative Medicine* (Berkeley: Celestial Arts, 2002).

39. Bland, Jeffrey S., Ph.D. and Sara H. Benum, M.A. *Genetic Nutritioneering* (Los Angeles: Keats, 1999).

40. Epstein, Samuel S., M.D. *The Politics of Cancer Revisited* (Hankins, NY: East Ridge Press, 1998).

41. Bland, *op cit.*

Chapter 5

1. Cancilla, Dorothy Rose. "The Medical Nightmare." *Townsend Letter for Doctors* 222 (January 2000):21.

2. Atkins, Robert C., M.D. *Dr. Atkins' New Diet Revolution* (New York: WholeCare/Avon, 2001).

3. Martin, Wayne. "Proteolytic Enzymes in Cancer Prevention and Treatment." *Townsend Letter for Doctors* 195 (October 1999):98–99.

4. Martin, *ibid.*

5. Spector, Michael. "The Outlaw Doctor." *New Yorker* 76(45) (Feb. 2001):48–61.

6. Simonton, O. Carl, M.D., Stephanie Matthews-Simonton, and James L. Creighton. *Getting Well Again* (New York: Bantam Books, 1978).

7. *ibid.*

8. Shippen, Eugene, M.D. and William Fryer. *The Testosterone Syndrome* (New York: Evans, 1998).

9. Wright, Jonathan, M.D. and Lane Lenard, Ph.D. *Maximize Your Vitality and Potency* (Petaluma: Smart Publications, 1999).

10. Zava, David, Ph.D. "Breast Cancer Risks." Your Own Health & Fitness, KPFA radio, March 2000.

11. Lee, John R., M.D. "Prostate Cancer." Address to the Prostate Awareness Foundation, San Francisco, CA, March 2000.

12. Shippen, *op cit.*

13. Lee, *op cit.*

14. Wright, *op cit.*

15. Wright, *op cit.*

16. Carruthers, Malcolm, M.D. *The Testosterone Revolution* (London: Thorsons, 2001).

17. Lee, *op cit* .

18. Peat, Ray, Ph.D. "Prostate Cancer." *Ray Peat's Newsletter* (May 1998):1–5.

19. Douglass, William Campbell, M.D. "CoQ10: An Amazing Cancer Treatment." *Second Opinion* (March 2000):5–23.

20. Wright, Jonathan, M.D. "Defeating out-of-control cell growth." *Life Enhancement* (Sept. 2000):5–23.

21. Rowen, Robert Jay, M.D. "Chinese Herb Cures Cancer." *Second Opinion* (May 2002):5–26.

22. Hoang, Ba, M.D., Ph.D., and Stephen Levine, Ph.D. "Botanical Therapies for Prostate Cancer." Address to the Prostate Awareness Foundation, Mill Valley, CA, May 2002.

23. www.rain-tree.com.

24. Lee, John R., M.D. "The Prostate Gland and Prostate Cancer." Address to the Institute of Health and Healing, San Francisco, June 2002.

25. www.poly-mva.com.

Chapter 6

1. Heiby, Walter A. *The Reverse Effect* (Deerfield, IL: MediScience Publishers, 1988).

2. Crayhon, Robert, M.S. *The Carntine Miracle* (New York: Evans, 1998).

3. Enig, Mary, Ph.D. *Know Your Fats* (Silver Spring, MD: Bethesda Press, 2000).

4. *ibid.*

5. *ibid.*

6. *ibid.*

7. Gerster, H. "Can adults adequately convert alpha-linoleic acid to EPA and DHA?" *International Journal of Vitamin and Nutrition Research* 68(1998):159–173.

8. Fallon, Sally. *Nourishing Traditions* (Washington, DC: New Trends, 1999).

9. Enig, *op cit.*

10. Allan, Christian B., Ph.D. "Life Without Bread." Your Own Health & Fitness, KPFA radio, May 2002.

11. Crayhon, *op cit.*

12. Andrew Weil, M.D. *Natural Health, Natural Medicine* (Boston: Houghton Mifflin, 1990).

13. Stoll, Andrew, M.D. *The Omega 3 Connection* (New York: Simon and Schuster, 2001).

14. Enig, *op cit.*

15. Heubeck, Elizabeth. "Dramatic evidence shows omega-3 fatty acids reduce risk of heart attack." *Life Extension* (July 2002):23.

16. Maillard, V. et al. "N-3 and N–6 fatty acids in breast adipose tissue and relative risk of breast cancer." *Intrnational Journal of Cancer* 98(1) (March 2002):78–83.

17. Howell, Edward. *Health and Longevity* (Woodstock Valley, CT: Omangod Press, 1980).

18. Pottenger, Francis M. Jr., M.D. *The Cat Studies* (San Diego: Price-Pottenger Nutrition Foundation, 1995).

19. Podmore, Ian, et al. "Vitamin C exhibits pro-oxidant properties." *Nature* 392 (April 9, 1998):559.

20. Podmore, Ian, et al. "Does vitamin C have a pro-oxidant effect?" *Nature* 395 (September 17, 1998):232.

21. Khaw, Kay-Tee, et al. "Relation between plasma ascorbic acid and mortality in men and women in EPIC-Norfolk prospective study." *The Lancet* 357 (March 3, 2001):657.

22. Weil, Andrew, M.D. "Vitamin C: A Change of Heart?" *Self Healing* (May 2000):5.

23. Cathcart, Robert, M.D. "The Ascorbate Effect in Viral Disease and Cancer." Address to the Orthomolecular Health-Medicine Society, San Francisco, CA, Feb. 2001.

24. Yudkin, John. *Sweet and Dangerous* (New York: Van Rees Press, 1972).

25. Crayhon, Robert, M.S. *Nutrition Made Simple* (New York: Evans, 1994).

26. DesMaisons, Kathleen, Ph.D. *Potatoes Not Prozac* (New York: Simon & Schuster, 1998).

27. Kreloff, Julie, M.S., R.D. "The Trouble with Fructose." *Designs for Health Weekly* (May 10, 2002): www.dfhi.com.

28. Hopkins, Virginia. "What about Sucralose?" *The John R. Lee, M.D. Medical Letter* (May 2002):4

29. Richard, David. *Stevia Rebaudiana: Nature's Sweet Secret* (Bloomingdale, IL: Vital Health Publishing, 1996).

30. Crayhon, Robert, M.S. and Julie Kreloff, M.S., R.D. "The Sweet Taste That's Good for You." *Designs for Health Weekly* (June 7, 2002): www.dfhi.com.

31. Hattersley, Joseph G., M.A. "The Nearest Thing to a Perfect Food: Part II." *Townsend Letter for Doctors* 227 (June 2002):86.

32. Fitzpatrick, Mike, Ph.D. "Soy: Panacea or Poison." Your Own Health & Fitness, KPFA radio, February 2000.

33. *ibid.*

34. Fallon, Sally, and Mary Enig, Ph.D. "Tragedy and Hope: The Third International Soy Symposium." *Townsend Letter for Doctors* 204 (July 2000):66–71.

Chapter 7

1. Morral, F.R. "Mercury: a historical review." *CIM Bulletin* (November 1984):81.

2. Svare, C.W. et al. "The effects of dental amalgams on mercury levels in expired air." *Journal of Dental Restoration* 60 (1981):1668–1671.

3. Vimy, M., Takahashi, Y., and Lorscheider, F.L. "Maternal-fetal distribution of mercury (203-Hg) released from dental amalgam fillings." *American Journal of Physiology* 258. (1990): R939–R945.

4. Kristal, Harold, J., D.D.S. "A study of the effects of mercury and nickel on the immune system." *Holistic Dental Journal* (April 1985):12–15.

5. Eggleston, David W., D.D.S. and Magnus Nylander, D.D.S. "Correlation of dental amalgam with mercury in brain tissue." *Journal of Prosthetic Dentistry* 58(6) (December 1987): 704–707.

6. Eggleston, David W., D.D.S. "Effect of dental amalgam and nickel alloy on T-lymphocytes." *Journal of Prosthetic Dentistry* 51(5) (1984): 627–623.

7. Bouquot, J. et al. "Neuralgia-inducing cavitational osteonecrosis." *Oral Surgery, Oral Medicine, Oral Pathology;* 73(3) (1992):07–319.

8. Waldbott, George L. *A Struggle With Titans* (New York: Carlton Press, 1965).

9. Coffel, Steve. "The Great Fluoride Fight." *Garbage* (May/June 1992):32–37.

Appendix A

1. Watson, George, Ph.D. *Nutrition and Your Mind* (New York: Harper and Row, 1972).

Bibliography

Metabolic Typing (Various Aspects)

Cousens, Gabriel, M.D. *Conscious Eating.* Berkeley: North Atlantic Books, 2000.

Garcia, Oz. *The Balance.* New York: Regan Books/HarperPerennial, 2000.

Kelley, William Donald, D.D.S. *The Metabolic Types.* Winthrop: Kelley Foundation, 1976.

Kelley, William Donald, D.D.S. *One Answer to Cancer.* Internet: Do-It-Yourself-Book, 1999.

Pottenger, Francis M., M.D. *Symptoms of Visceral Disease.* St. Louis: C.V. Mosby, 1944.

Schenker, Guy R., D.C. *An Analytical System of Clinical Nutrition.* Mifflintown, PA: Nutri-Spec, 1999.

Watson, George, Ph.D. *Nutrition and Your Mind.* New York: Harper and Row, 1972.

Wiley, Rudolf A., Ph.D. *BioBalance.* Hurricane, UT: Essential Science Publishing, 1998.

Wolcott, William L., and Trish Fahey. *The Metabolic Typing Diet.* New York: Doubleday, 2000.

Cancer

Ausubel, Kenny. *When Healing Became a Crime.* Rochester: Healing Arts Press, 2000.

Epstein, Samuel S., M.D. *The Politics of Cancer Revisited.* Hankins, NY: East Ridge Press, 1998.

Epstein, Samuel S., M.D. *The Breast Cancer Prevention Program.* New York: Hungry Minds 1996.

Lee, John R., M.D., David Zava, Ph.D., and Virginia Hopkins. *What Your Doctor May Not Tell You about Breast Cancer.* New York: Warner, 2002.

Simonton, O. Carl, M.D., Stephanie Matthews-Simonton, and James L. Creighton. *Getting Well Again.* New York: Bantam Books, 1978.

Heart Health

Bayan, Matthew J. *Eat Fat, Be Healthy.* New York: Fireside/Simon and Schuster, 2000.

McCully, Kilmer, M.D. *The Homocysteine Revolution.* Los Angeles: Keats, 1997.

Ravnskov, Uffe, M.D., Ph.D. *The Cholesterol Myths.* Washington, DC: New Trends Publishing, 2000.

Reaven, Gerald M., M.D. *Syndrome X: The Silent Killer.* New York: Fireside/Simon and Schuster, 2000.

Wayne, Howard, M.D. *How to Protect Your Heart from Your Doctor.* Santa Barbara: Capra Press, 1994.

Hormones

Carruthers, Malcolm, M.D. *The Testosterone Revolution.* London: Thorsons, 2001.

Lee, John R., M.D., and Virginia Hopkins. *What Your Doctor May Not Tell You about Menopause.* New York: Warner, 1996.

Lee, John R., M.D., Jesse Hanley, M.D., and Virginia Hopkins. *What Your Doctor May Not Tell You About Premenopause*. New York: Warner, 1999.

Shames, Richard L., M.D. *Thyroid Power: 10 Steps to Total Health*. New York: Quill/Harper Collins, 2002.

Shippen, Eugene, M.D., and William Fryer. *The Testosterone Syndrome*. New York: Evans, 1998.

Wilson, James L., N.D., D.C., Ph.D. *Adrenal Fatigue: The 21st Century Stress Syndrome*. Petaluma: Smart Publications, 2001.

Wright, Jonathan, M.D., and Lane Lenard, Ph.D. *Maximize Your Vitality and Potency*. Petaluma: Smart Publications, 1999.

Miscellaneous

Abravanel, Elliot D., M.D. *Dr. Abravanel's Body Type Diet and Lifestyle Nutrition Plan*. New York: Bantam Books, 1999.

Allan, Christian B., Ph.D. and Wolfgang Lutz, M.D. *Life Without Bread*. Los Angeles: Keats, 2000.

Atkins, Robert C., M.D. *Dr. Atkins' New Diet Revolution*. New York: WholeCare/Avon, 2001.

Balch, Phyllis, C.N.C., and James F. Balch, M.D. *Prescription for Nutritional Healing*. New York: Avery, 2000.

Bernstein, Richard K., M.D. *Dr. Bernstein's Diabetes Solution*. New York: Little Brown, 1997.

Bland, Jeffrey S., Ph.D., and Sara H. Benum, M.A. *Genetic Nutritioneering*. Los Angeles: Keats, 1999.

Braverman, Eric. R., M.D. *The Healing Nutrients Within*. Los Angeles: Keats, 1997.

Cheraskin, Emmanuel, D.D.S., and W. M. Ringsdorf, D.D.S. *Predictive Medicine: A Study in Strategy*. Mountain View, CA: Pacific Press, 1973.

Cordain, Loren, Ph.D. *The Paleo Diet*. New York: Wiley, 2002.

Crayhon, Robert, M.S. *The Carnitine Miracle*. New York: Evans, 1998.

———*Nutrition Made Simple*. New York: Evans, 1994.

D'Adamo, Peter , Ph.D. *Eat Right for Your Type*. New York: Putnam, 1997.

Davis, Adelle. *Let's Eat Right to Keep Fit*. New York: Harcourt Brace, 1954.

———*You Can Get Well*. New York: Poor Boy Press, 1975.

DesMaisons, Kathleen, Ph.D. *Potatoes Not Prozac*. New York: Simon & Schuster, 1998.

Dispenza, Joseph. *Live Better Longer*. New York: Harper Collins, 1997.

Eades, Michael R., MD., and Mary Dan Eades, M.D. *Protein Power*. New York: Bantam, 1996.

Enig, Mary, Ph.D. *Know Your Fats*. Silver Spring, MD: Bethesda Press, 2000.

Erdmann, Robert, Ph.D. *The Amino Revolution*. New York: Simon & Schuster, 1989.

Fallon, Sally. *Nourishing Traditions: The Cookbook That Challenges Politically Correct Nutrition and the Diet Dictocrats*. Washington, DC: New Trends, 1999.

Galland, Leo, M.D. *Power Healing*. New York: Random House, 1997.

Goldberg, Burton. *Alternative Medicine*. Berkeley: Celestial Arts, 2002.

Gottschall, Elaine, B.A., M.Sc. *Breaking the Vicious Cycle*. Baltimore: The Kirkton Press, 1998.

Heiby, Walter A. *The Reverse Effect*. Deerfield, IL: MediScience Publishers, 1988.

Huggins, Hal, D.D.S. *Uninformed Consent: The Hidden Dangers in Dental Care*. Charlottesville: Hampton Roads, 1998.

Lininger, Schuyler W., Jr., D.C., editor. *A-Z Guide to Drug-Herb-Vitamin Interactions*. Rocklin: Prima, 1999.

Lipski, Elizabeth, M.S., C.C.N. *Digestive Wellness*. Los Angeles: Keats, 2000.

Mondoa, Emil I., M.D., and Mindy Kitei. *Sugars That Heal: The New Healing Science of Glyconutrients.* New York: Ballantine, 2001.

Murray, Michael, N.D., and Joseph Pizzorno, N.D. *Encyclopedia of Natural Medicine.* Rocklin, CA: Prima, 1998.

Perlmutter, David, M.D. *BrainRecovery.com.* Naples, FL: Perlmutter Health Center, 2000.

Pottenger, Francis M. Jr., M.D. *The Cat Studies.* San Diego: Price-Pottenger Nutrition Foundation, 1995.

Price, Weston A., D.D.S. *Nutrition and Physical Degeneration.* Los Angeles: Keats, 1989.

Ross, Julia, M.A. The Diet Cure. New York: Viking, 1999.

Sears, Barry, Ph.D., and Bill Lawren. *The Zone.* New York: Harper Collins, 1995.

Schmid, Ronald, N.D. *Traditional Foods Are Your Best Medicine.* Rochester: Healing Arts Press, 1997.

Selye, Hans , M.D. *Stress Without Distress.* New York: Signet, 1974.

Siegel, Bernie S., M.D. *Love, Medicine & Miracles.* New York: HarperPerennial, 1998.

Watts, David. L., D.C., Ph.D. *Trace Elements and Other Essential Nutrients.* Addison, TX: Trace Elements, 1997.

Williams, Roger J., Ph.D. *Nutrition Against Disease.* New York: Bantam Books, 1978.

Index

About the Authors

HAROLD J. KRISTAL, D.D.S.

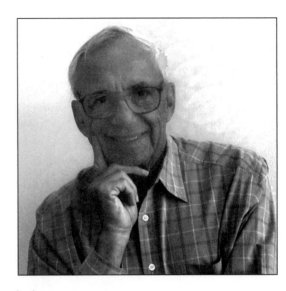

Harold J. Kristal graduated from the University of Minnesota School of Dentistry in 1947. He moved to California, joined the Navy for one year as a dentist, later transferring to the Air Force for two more years, holding the rank of captain. Subsequently he was in private practice in Richmond and Point Richmond, California until 1993. He has been a member of American Dental Association for forty-eight years, a Fellow in the American Institute of Oral Biology, and is a past President of the Contra Costa Dental Association.

Over time, Dr. Kristal came to question the use of mercury in dental amalgams, as well as the safety of several other mainstream dental practices. He became one of the pioneers in the new holistic (or biological) dentistry movement and, from 1983–89, he was Chairman of the University of California Holistic Dental Study Club. During this time he arranged for several guest speakers to lecture to the study group, many of whom were prominent people in the world of alternative health. Guest lecturers in this series included John R. Lee, M.D., Parris Kidd, Ph.D., Michael Rosenbaum, M.D., and Jeffrey Bland, Ph.D. During this time he also presented two-day nutritional seminars, from Hawaii to New York, while also appearing as a guest speaker on Dr. Jeffrey Bland's highly regarded metabolic update tape series.

Throughout this period, Dr. Kristal's long-held belief in the connection between dental health and the health of the whole body was affirmed, as well as his conviction of the importance of sound nutrition. Throughout much of his career as a dentist, he incorporated nutritional counseling into his practice, experimenting over the years with various different systems of nutritional analysis. In 1993 he retired from his dental practice, moving full-time into the practice of nutritional counseling. He worked extensively at a distance with William Wolcott, the original synthesizer of the integrated form of Metabolic Typing, over a period of several years, to further refine the testing and interpretation protocols of Metabolic Typing. Dr. Kristal was especially instrumental in developing the in-office testing procedures used by practitioners of Metabolic Typing.

Dr. Kristal maintains a busy Metabolic Typing practice at Metabolic Nutrition, his nutrition clinic in San Rafael, California. He also teaches several Metabolic Typing seminars each year to health professionals, both in the US. and in Europe, has been interviewed on several radio and television shows, and has spoken before various health groups. He has also published numerous articles on nutrition and Metabolic Typing in such publications as the *Townsend Letter for Doctors* and *Alternative Medicine.*

JAMES M. HAIG, N.C.

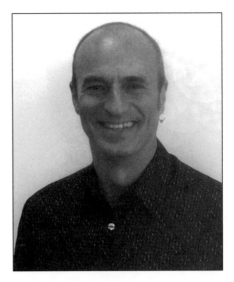

A long-time student of nutrition and health trends, James M. Haig, B.A. Hons., N.C. is a nutritionist, health educator, and health writer living and working in Marin County, California. He is an alumnus of the University of Leicester, England, from which he graduated with a B.A. Honors in Combined Arts, and the Institute of Educational Therapy (IET) in Cotati, California, from which he graduated Magna Cum Laude as a Nutrition Consultant. For many years James worked in the music business, rising to the position of Vice President of Sales and Operations for a wholesale distribution company. He has also worked for nutritional supplement companies in various capacities, including research, writing, editing, customer support, and marketing. He has studied and practiced Metabolic Typing with Dr. Harold J. Kristal since 1998, and assists him in teaching Personalized Metabolic Nutrition Seminars to medical doctors and other health professionals; he also edited and co-wrote the *Personalized Metabolic Nutrition Practitioners' Manual.* James has co-authored articles that have appeared in the *Townsend Letter for Doctors, Alternative Medicine, Health and Healing Wisdom* (the journal of the Price-Pottenger Nutrition Foundation) and *The Communicator* (the journal of the Holistic Dental Association), and he is the founder and editor of the bimonthly newsletter *Metabolic News.* When not involved with his nutritional pursuits, James likes to get lost in the hills near his home in Northern California.

North Atlantic Books Series:
Food as Medicine, Food as Consciousness

North Atlantic Books has developed a series of unique books on food as medicine and the relationship between diet and consciousness. These books transcend traditional categories of nutrition, alternative medicine, and spiritual practice to discuss health, diet, and consumption in terms of our actual human situation. The three titles presently comprising the series are *Healing with Whole Foods: Asian Traditions and Modern Nutrition* by Paul Pitchford (published originally in 1993; revised and updated in 2002); *Conscious Eating* by Gabriel Cousens, M.D. (published originally by Essene Vision Books in 1992; enlarged, revised, and republished by North Atlantic Books in 2000); and *How We Heal: Nutritional, Emotional, and Psychospiritual Fundamentals* by Douglas Morrison (published originally by Health Hope Publishing House as *Body Electronics Fundamentals* in 1993; enlarged, revised, and republished by North Atlantic Books in 2001). A fourth title, *Everyday Vegan* by Jeani-Rose Atchison, is a cookbook written in the spirit of conscious diet.

These books propose that every food is a medicine (and has long-term secondary effects on both our organs and our psyche) and that each medicine is likewise a food (and directly affects metabolic balance and energetic capacity).

In all three "food as medicine, food as consciousness" books, consumption is viewed not just as a mechanical event of nutrition and bodily maintenance nor as sensual recreation but also as a total psychospiritual process. Dietary sources and preparation, cooking procedures and utensils, levels of taste and consumption awareness, and diverse facets of digestion and fasting are explored. The authors are concerned with the assimilation and transmutation of what enters the body-mind (including enzymes, minerals, oils, type of water, type of air, etc.) rather than what is either enjoyable and pleasing to consume or rumored to be healthy. Each of these books explores the deeper cellular satisfaction and resonance that come from eating, drinking, and combining foods as part of a serious daily practice. Each ask: what makes food alive?; how does eating teach you who you are?; how can whole foods and conscious eating help you find your destiny?

Each of the books also deals with the impact human beings have on the Earth and its sentient beings (the role of compassion and responsibility in diet), plus the reciprocal effects of the planet's environment on health and food. They presume that eating must be attuned to communities and ecosystems.

Note: These books were written independently of one another. The individual authors' advice, while overlapping in some areas, disagrees in others, sometimes even offering contradictory solutions to the same issues (for instance, the advantages and drawbacks of cooking and consuming food raw). None of the authors specifically recommends the other two books or has any connection to them.

North Atlantic Books as a publisher is presenting these separate visions for readers to consider in creating their own diets and addressing their own self-healing. Individuals will find ideas in one or another book better suited to their own constitutions and temperaments, so every reader should use sound personal judgment and intuition in choosing a path of food.

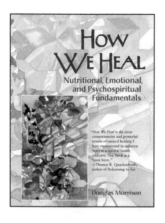

How We Heal:
Nutritional, Emotional, and Psychospiritual Fundamentals

By Douglas Morrison
ISBN: 1-55643-362-X
$27.50 trade paper, 488 pp.
illustrations

"... for healing to be possible, we must desire this healing and yet have no attachment to it: we must remain willing to not heal. We must be willing to put our full effort into the process and yet have no attachment to the outcome of that effort." —from the book

This book addresses healing in the broadest conceivable context. Though *How We Heal* is a comprehensive resource on the physical basis of health, it goes far beyond the physical to examine the emotional and spiritual elements that cause illness and can block even the most powerful healing methods from success. Morrison's genius lies in explaining the full nature of the healing crisis and the role of resistance in preventing us from getting well. This book serves as an excellent introduction to the frontiers of healing, where the most advanced realms of molecular science meet the most esoteric aspects of spirit.

How We Heal explores some of the more cutting-edge methods of diagnosis and healing, including iridology, sclerology, and Body Electronics. An extensive section on nutrition includes cooking methods, the research of Dr. Weston A. Price, diet versus supplements, digestion, elimination, the role of friendly microbes within our digestive system, and the use of probiotics. Topics such as sleep, air and breathing, quantity and quality of water, exercise methods, bodywork techniques, and the dangers of amalgam dental fillings, root canals, fluoride, electromagnetic fields, vaccinations, drugs, and tobacco are considered in a clear, informative way. Yet, as thoroughly as Morrison presents all these physical factors, the author never loses sight of the much larger picture, and it is his ability to integrate the physical, emotional, mental, and spiritual aspects of health that is truly at the heart of this book.

Douglas Morrison studied Body Electronics with its founder, Dr. John Whitman Ray, and has been teaching seminars since 1988. He is a graduate of Harvard University and holds doctorate degrees in naturopathy, nutritional counseling, and alternative medicine.

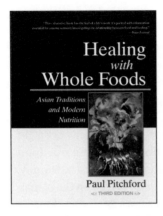

Healing with Whole Foods:
Asian Traditions and Modern Nutrition

By Paul Pitchford
ISBN: 1-55643-220-8
$35.00 trade paper, 730 pp.
charts, diagrams, illustrations

Paul Pitchford's *Healing with Whole Foods* is acknowledged internationally as the authoritative source of integrative and client-specific nutrition. Unique in the history of books on food and diet, this work merges modern nutrition with insight from ancient Asian traditions. More than seven hundred pages provide life-enhancing guidelines to renewal and rejuvenation, allowing the reader to develop an optimal diet to fit his or her constitutional type.

This comprehensive reference work features:

- current guidelines on nutrition basics, such as the protein/vitamin B_{12} group, fats and oils, sugars and sweeteners, water, salt, seaweeds, "green foods" (micro-algae and cereal grasses), calcium, oxygen, and other nutritional items.

- clear discussions of the Chinese healing arts applied to physical and emotional conditions, including the Eight Principles (Six Divisions of Yin and Yang), Five Elements, and syndromes of the internal organs.

- information on making a gentle transition from an animal-products-based diet to one centered on whole grains and fresh vegetables; there are over three hundred healthful vegan recipes presented, as well as detailed information on the healing properties of plant and animal foods.

- sections on weight loss, heart and vascular renewal, female health, digestive problems, candida yeast infections, root canals, food combining, fasting, children, pregnancy, and aging; includes insights from Ayurvedic medicine of India.

- detailed "regeneration diets" and herbal treatments for cancer, arthritis, mental illness, drug and alcohol abuse, AIDS, and other degenerative conditions; also features a "parasite purge program" tailored to specific body types.

Paul Pitchford is a healer, teacher, and nutrition researcher. He has taught at various learning centers, including universities and schools of East Asian medicine, and lectured at numerous healing events. Pitchford currently lives in Northern California, where he directs the Heartwood Institute Wellness Clinic and Oriental Healing Arts Program, located in Garberville, CA.

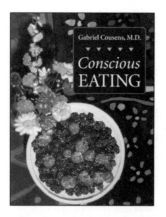

Conscious Eating

By Gabriel Cousens, M.D.
ISBN: 1-55643-285-2
$35.00 trade paper, 874 pp.
illustrations, charts, recipes

Long viewed as the bible of vegetarianism, *Conscious Eating* is a comprehensive effort to bring clarity and light to the most essential questions regarding our food choices and the process of living healthfully, happily, and in increased harmony with all beings on the planet.

Conscious Eating not only serves as an encyclopedia of vegetarian, vegan, live-food, and organic nutrition, but is really four books in one: Principles of Individualizing the Diet; The Choice of Vegetarianism; Transition to Vegetarianism and Live-Foods; and The Art of Live-Food Preparation. The mystery and mastery of *Conscious Eating* is that it integrates all four books into one. Read one book at a time, the entire text, or use it as a reference.

Conscious Eating, in a revolutionary approach, addresses the uniqueness of each human and empowers readers to deal with this scientific reality as opposed to the "one diet serves all" approach of fad books. Readers will learn how to individualize their diets for their particular psycho-physiological types—including four main perspectives: fast/slow oxidizer; parasympathetic/sympathetic autonomic; ayurvedic; and blood type—to optimize their health on all levels.

Explore chapter after chapter of new information including:
- How to heal the "biologically-altered brain"—the result of genetic weakness compounded by generations of poor diet and present poor diet combined with environmental and emotional toxicities.
- A mind-body-spirit approach to the vegetarian way of life.
- The importance of vegetarianism in healing self and ecology of the planet.
- The most complete scientific explanation of vegetarianism and vitamin B_{12}.
- Live-food and nutrition: from biophysics to metaphysics.
- An extensive chapter on enzymes—the secret of health and longevity.
- New theory of nutrition: why the material/mechanistic theory of nutrition (nutrition focusing on calories) is inadequate, misleading, and an inaccurate way of understanding nutrition.
- The art of live-food preparation: two hundred recipes included.
- In-depth discussion on the transition to vegetarianism, veganism, and live-foods.

Gabriel Cousens, M.D. and Diplomat of Ayurveda, is one of the foremost medical proponents of a vegetarian/vegan, live-food, one-hundred-percent organic diet as a key component to maximum health and spiritual awareness. He is the founder/director of the Tree of Life Rejuvenation Center located in Patagonia, Arizona.